ICU Manual for Nurses

ICU Manual for Nurses

Prakash Shastri MD FRCA (UK) FICCM
Vice-Chairmam
Department of Critical Care and Emergency Medicine
Sir Ganga Ram Hospital
New Delhi, India

Forewords
BK Rao
Shirish Prayag

JAYPEE

JAYPEE BROTHERS MEDICAL PUBLISHERS
The Health Sciences Publisher
New Delhi | London

JAYPEE **Jaypee Brothers Medical Publishers (P) Ltd**

Headquarters
EMCA House
23/23-B, Ansari Road, Daryaganj
New Delhi - 110 002, India
Landline: +91-11-23272143, +91-11-23272703
+91-11-23282021, +91-11-23245672
E-mail: jaypee@jaypeebrothers.com

Corporate Office
4838/24, Ansari Road, Daryaganj
New Delhi - 110 002, India
Phone: +91-11-43574357
Fax: +91-11-43574314
E-mail: jaypee@jaypeebrothers.com

Overseas Office
J.P. Medical Ltd
83 Victoria Street, London
SW1H 0HW (UK)
Phone: +44 20 3170 8910
E-mail: info@jpmedpub.com

EU GPSR Authorised Representative
Logos Europe, 9 rue Nicolas Poussin
17000, La Rochelle, France
Phone: +33 (0) 6 67 93 73 78
E-mail: contact@logoseurope.eu

Website: www.jaypeebrothers.com
Website: www.jaypeedigital.com

Inquiries for bulk sales may be solicited at: jaypee@jaypeebrothers.com

ICU Manual for Nurses

First Edition: **2017**

Reprint: **2026**

ISBN: 978-93-86322-96-8

Printed at: Samrat Offset Pvt. Ltd.

Contributors

Anna George BDS MHM PGDMLE
General Manager
Department of Quality Assurance
Rajagiri Hospital
Aluva, Kerala, India

Bhanu P Zawar MD FIACTA
Associate Consultant
Institute of Anesthesiology and Critical Care
Medanta - The Medicity
Gurugram, Haryana, India

Debashish Dhar MD
Senior Consultant
Department of Critical Care and Emergency Medicine
Sir Ganga Ram Hospital
New Delhi, India

Deepak Govil MD EDIC
Associate Director
Institute of Anesthesiology and Critical Care
Medanta - The Medicity
Gurugram, Haryana, India

Disha Magatpalli MD MBA
Senior Consultant
Apollo Hospital
Visakhapatnam, Andhra Pradesh, India

Judith Vasan MSc (Medical Surgical Nursing)
Chief Nursing Officer
Global Hospital
Hyderabad, Telangana, India

Jyoti Randhawa MBBS MBA (Operation Management)
PGD (Medical Law and Ethics) PGDBM (NIHFW) DMS
Sir Ganga Ram Hospital
New Delhi, India

Kapil Zirpe MD FICCM FCCM
Director and Head
Department of Neurotrauma
Grant Medical Foundation
Ruby Hall Clinic
Pune, Maharashtra, India

Lawni Goswami MD EDIC
Consultant Critical Care
Apollo Gleneagles Hospitals
Kolkata, West Bengal, India

Mahuya Bhattacharyya MD IDCC FNB (Critical Care)
Consultant Critical Care
AMRI Hospital
Kolkata, West Bengal, India

Manish Munjal MD FICCM FCCS PFCCS
Member Editorial Board
Indian Journal of Critical Care Medicine
Member Secretary
Indian College of Critical Care Medicine
Chairman, Jigyasa Foundation
Jaipur, Rajasthan, India

Mohan Maharaj MD MBA IDCC PDCC
Medical Director
Care Hospital
Visakhapatnam, Andhra Pradesh, India

Navneet Mehta MD
Director and Head
Department of Cardiac Anesthesia and Cardiac Critical Care
Eternal Hospital
Jaipur, Rajasthan, India

Pradeep D'Costa DNB IDCC
Consultant Intensivist
KEM and Sahyadri Hospital
Pune, Maharashtra, India

Prajakta Samir Hindlekar RN MSN
Director Nursing
Breach Candy Hospital Trust
Mumbai, Maharashtra, India

Prakash Shastri MD FRCA (UK) FICCM
Vice-Chairmam
Department of Critical Care and Emergency Medicine
Sir Ganga Ram Hospital
New Delhi, India

Praveen Venishetty DTCD DNB (Respiratory Medicine)
Senior Registrar
Apollo Main Hospital
Chennai, Tamil Nadu, India

Rajesh Mohan Shetty FRCA(UK) FFICM(UK) FCICM(Aus and Nz)
Consultant Intensivist and Medical Superintendent
Manipal Hospital
Bengaluru, Karnataka, India

Raymond D Savio MD DM EDIC
Consultant, Critical Care Medicine
Apollo Main Hospital
Chennai, Tamil Nadu, India

RK Mani MD MRCP (UK) FCCP
Group CEO
Nayati Super Speciality Hospital
Chairman, Critical Care and Pulmonology
Mathura, Uttar Pradesh, India

Sanjay MV MD FIPA FNF EDIC
Junior Consultant (Critical Care Medicine)
Apollo Main Hospital
Chennai, Tamil Nadu, India

Sharanappa GNM PGDCR PBBSc (Nursing)
Senior Staff Nurse and ICU Clinical Educator
Manipal Hospital
Bengaluru, Karnataka, India

Shilpi Khanna DNB (Microbiology)
Head
Department of Microbiology and CSSD
Mata Chanan Devi Hospital
New Delhi, India

Subhash Todi MD MRCP
Senior Consultant
Critical Care and Emergency Medicine
AMRI Hospital
Kolkata, West Bengal, India

Supradip Ghosh DNB (Internal Medicine) MNAMS EDIC
Consultant and Head, Critical Care Medicine
Fortis-Escorts Hospitals
Faridabad, Haryana, India

Sushma Gurav DNB (Anesthetia) IDCCM
Consultant, Neurotrauma Unit
Grant Medical Foundation
Ruby Hall Clinic
Pune, Maharashtra, India

Vajrapu Rajendra MD (NIMS) FNB (SGRH N. Delhi) EDIC(UK)
Senior Consultant, Critical Care and Incharge MICU
Head of the Department of Critical Care and Internal Medicine
Aware Global Hospitals
Hyderabad, Telangana, India

Vasudha Sethi MPT (Musculoskeletal)
Physiotherapist (ICU)
Sir Ganga Ram Hospital
New Delhi, India

Vinod Singh MD MRCP EDIC
Senior Consultant
Department of Critical Care and Emergency Medicine
Sir Ganga Ram Hospital
New Delhi, India

Vitrag Shah MD (Med)
FNB Fellow
Department of Critical Care and Emergency Medicine
Sir Ganga Ram Hospital
New Delhi, India

Yatin Mehta MD FRCA
Director
Institute of Anesthesiology and Critical Care
Medanta - The Medicity
Gurugram, Haryana, India

Foreword

It gives me a great pleasure to write the foreword for the book *ICU Manual for Nurses*. The book has nine sections covering from the essentials of patient care like assessment, infections, mechanical ventilation and monitoring to the specialty nursing. The format of the book is easy-to-read and understand. The information contained in the chapters is well structured and presented in a clear, concise and stepwise fashion.

There are not sufficient books written keeping Indian critical care nursing needs in mind. I congratulate the authors who have contributed to the contents of the book. I hope this handbook will serve as a reference guide to the beginners as well as practising critical care nurses.

BK Rao MD
Chairman,
Department of Critical Care and Emergency Medicine
Sir Ganga Ram Hospital
New Delhi, India

Foreword

I feel a great pride and pleasure to write this foreword for the book of *ICU Manual for Nurses*.

Nurses form perhaps the most important component of the team which cares for the Critically Ill patients. They are constantly with the patients, and their constant vigil as well as actions go a long way in the contribution to the effort to save the life of a critically ill patients.

Intensive care has come a long way since the era when caring nurses and doctors looked after the really sick patients in a section of the hospital. We now have an array of equipment and the science of treating these patients, and this has evolved to become a full fledged speciality. As a result, all those who work in the field of critical care need a sound knowledge of the theory and practice.

This training involves reading material as well as bedside practice. There is a huge amount of material available for training doctors in this field. However, in India, the training of nurses has lagged far behind the training of doctors. The Indian Society of Critical Care Medicine [ISCCM] has recognized this deficiency and has been conducting the training programs for nurses. Amongst the office bearers of ISCCM who have strived hard to cover this lacuna, the name of Dr Prakash Shastri stands first. He has been amongst the few who have consistently attempted to systematically train the nurses in this specialty.

The result of all his hard work has been showcased in this book. It covers all the important areas which the ICU nurses need to be taught, from theory to practice, and from ventilators and other machines to the infection control measures like handwashing and others. All these chapters have been written with scientifically accurate language, and it is still easy to read because of the lucidity.

Dr Prakash Shastri and all the coauthors deserve a lot of kudos for coming out with this book, through their patience and hard work. It is a must read for all nurses who are training in intensive care and also a must for the ICU nurses room tables.

I wish all the best for this book and hope that it will add to the competence of ICU nurses and contribute significantly to the saving of lives which we all attempt in ICUs.

Shirish Prayag MD FCCM
Past President and Founder Executive Member, ISCCM
Past Editor, IJCCM
Shree Medical Foundation Prayag Hospital
Pune, Maharastra, India

Preface

Critical care nursing has grown as a specialty around the world. However, in many regions, there is still an urgent need for professional education to improve the outcome of patient suffering from life-threatening illness. Critical care nurses work in settings where patients require complex assessment, high intensity therapies, interventions, and continuous vigilance. They need specialized knowledge, skills and experience to provide care to the patients.

The contribution of nurses toward achieving the goals in critical care is equal to any other healthcare professionals, if not more. In recognizing the responsibility of nurses in ICU, the Indian Society of Critical Care Medicine has started the Indian Diploma in Critical Care Nursing course. This manual intends to meet the needs of this course.

Prakash Shastri

Contents

Section 1: Introduction
Prakash Shastri

1. **ICU Nursing—How is it Different?** 3
Prakash Shastri

Section 2: Fundamentals of ICU Care
Prakash Shastri

2. **Airway Management** 9
Debashish Dhar

3. **Oral Care** 15
Prajakta Samir Hindlekar

4. **Eye Care** 19
Prajakta Samir Hindlekar

5. **Pressure Sores** 23
Prajakta Samir Hindlekar

6. **Physiotherapy in Intensive Care Unit** 28
Vasudha Sethi

7. **Fast Hugs Bid** 31
Sanjay MV, Raymond D Savio

8. **Delirium in the Intensive Care Unit** 42
Praveen Venishetty, Raymond D Savio

9. **Sedation in the Critically Ill** 50
Raymond D Savio

Section 3: Patient Monitoring
Supradip Ghosh

10. **Hemodynamics in Critical Care** 57
Supradip Ghosh

11. **Pulse Oximetry and End-tidal Carbon Dioxide Monitoring** 67
Supradip Ghosh

Section 4: Mechanical Ventilation
Vinod Singh

12. **Basics of Mechanical Ventilation** 73
Vinod Singh, Vitrag Shah

13. Noninvasive Ventilation 82
Vinod Singh

Section 5: Fluids and Transfusion Therapy
Subhash Todi

14. Fluid Replacement Therapy 87
Mohan Maharaj, Disha Magatpalli

15. Blood and Blood Products 93
Mohan Maharaj, Disha Magatpalli

16. Nutritional Support in Critical Care 98
Subhash Todi, Mahuya Bhattacharyya

Section 6: Infection
Rajesh Mohan Shetty

17. Infection Control and the ICU Bundles 107
Rajesh Mohan Shetty, Sharanappa

Section 7: Speciality Nursing
Yatin Mehta

18. Cardiac Critical Care 125
Yatin Mehta, Bhanu P Zawar

19. Postoperative Care of Coronary Artery Bypass Graft Patients 136
Manish Munjal, Navneet Mehta

20. Neurocritical Care 141
Kapil Zirpe, Sushma Gurav

21. Liver Failure 151
Deepak Govil

22. Acute Renal Failure in Intensive Care Unit and Renal Replacement Therapy 157
Pradeep D'Costa

Section 8: Miscellaneous
Prakash Shastri

23. Sampling for Investigations in Critically-ill Patients 163
Shilpi Khanna

24. Needlestick Injury 174
Lawni Goswami

25. Sterilization and Waste Management 179
Jyoti Randhawa

26. Nursing Communication in Intensive Care Units **189**
Anna George, Raymond D Savio

27. Documentation in Intensive Care Unit **197**
Judith Vasan, Vajrapu Rajendra

28. Defibrillation and Cardioversion **221**
Vajrapu Rajendra, Judith Vasan

29. Terminal Care of a Dying Patient **224**
RK Mani

Appendix *227*

Index *231*

Section 1

Introduction

SECTION EDITOR: Prakash Shastri

1

CHAPTER

ICU Nursing—How is it Different?

Prakash Shastri

The difference in the ICU is that health care personnel are working under a constant threat to life. The stress levels are high and responses need to be immediate. Maintaining a constant high standard of intensive care is the greatest challenge for an ICU. The nursing staff is the mainstay in achieving that goal. They are responsible for most of the minute-to-minute monitoring and treatment. In addition to conventional nursing responsibilities, much of the clinical decision making can be decentralized to a skilled nursing staff. This requires investment in teaching, in service programs and audits directed at the bedside nurse.

The permanent senior medical and nursing staff must provide the continuity of care and ensure that standards are maintained within an ICU. They are responsible for the orientation, education and training of new staff. Junior medical staff usually rotate through the ICU for varying periods and this can lead to inconsistency in the care of patients unless standardization is ensured through protocols, supervision and educational programs.

EXPANDED ROLE OF NURSES

Weaning

The weaning process (e.g. adjusting ventilatory rates and pressures) can be carried out by the nursing staff using laboratory data and bedside monitoring.

Drugs

Inotropes, vasodilators, sedatives, analgesics, insulin and many other drugs can be given by continuous intravenous (IV) infusion. Adjustments of infusion rates can be decided by nursing staff, based on clinical and laboratory data.

Infection Control

The entire gamut of processes and protocols involving infection control in the ICU revolves around the nurse.

OTHER ASPECTS OF WARD FUNCTION

The nursing staff should be integrated into all aspects of administration of the ICU, in addition to taking care of the patients and dealing with their friends and relatives. Other members of the intensive care staff may include physiotherapists, ward clerks, social workers and ward attendants. They are all essential for an efficiently run team. Although it is difficult to measure the effect on patient outcome of a well-organized team, most experienced intensivists value this aspect of their unit highly and invest time and energy in achieving it.

Ward Rounds and Continuity

There should be at least one comprehensive ward round each day. The half-life of major decisions regarding seriously ill patients is approximately 24 hours, whereas for patients in general wards it is approximately 3–4 days. The medical staff, nursing staff and others involved in a patient's management should formulate a strategy for the next 24 hours. This is a framework around which fine-tuning can occur, depending on changes in the patient's condition and the findings on laboratory tests. Like other strategies, it must be flexible enough to allow changes according to the patient's condition. Rather than using a system that features a provisional diagnosis and final diagnosis, one must take a problem-orientated approach to seriously ill patients.

Detailed handovers with a short- and long-term plan are essential for continuity and optimal management of the patient, especially by senior medical staff.

Relatives and Friends

The condition of a patient should be explained in an honest and forthright manner to relatives and friends. There is no place for false hope and avoidance of difficult explanations—even if it means admitting that many aspects of the patient's disease process are, as yet, unknown. It helps to have a special information pamphlet for the patient's friends and relatives that will explain certain matters such as:

- Relevant aspects of the hospital's function.
- Visiting policy for the ICU.
- The invasive lines and machines that may be encountered.

Labeled photographs of the various pieces of equipment and lines, with a short description of each, can be displayed in the waiting room.

An explanation of the possible time course of the patient's illness must be given. Many relatives wish to maintain an all-night vigil during the early part of a critical illness, when the patient conceivably could remain stable for days or weeks. It is important to inform relatives of such possibilities so that they can arrange their schedules regarding sleep, work and other responsibilities.

QUALITY ASSURANCE

Quality assurance (QA), auditing and peer review are all concepts that generally have to do with monitoring and attempting to improve current practice. The idea behind most efforts in this area is that practitioners can demonstrate to themselves and to others the quality and quantity of work they are doing. The principles of QA and total quality management (TQM) readily lend themselves to managing an ICU.

Decision making and autonomy must be decentralized to the bedside. The ability to make decisions comes through education. Making changes is difficult, and many who have been trained in a different way will feel uncomfortable. We need, ultimately, to reach the point at which we begin to feel comfortable with many of the unpredictable aspects of our practice, until eventually we can thrive on the non-routine.

The staff need to be encouraged to be autonomous and to speak out when the system is not working. Senseless rules need to be eliminated. The common good should always be put above one's own. This system will not be the place for large egos that are easily bruised.

2
Section

Fundamentals of ICU Care

SECTION EDITOR: Prakash Shastri

2

CHAPTER

Airway Management

Debashish Dhar

Emergency management universally starts with management of A-B-C, i.e. airway; breathing and circulation. The cornerstone of airway management of any critically ill patient is to ensure oxygenation.

Airway acts as a conduit for the ambient air to reach the lungs during breathing. Airway is divided into two parts: upper and lower and they comprise following anatomical parts:

- Upper airway: Nose, mouth, pharynx and larynx (till glottic opening).
- Lower airway: Subglottic larynx, trachea, bronchi and bronchioles.

Upper airway is roughly what is visualized by laryngoscopy. Airway is just the passage through which air passes and has no role in gas exchange. But it is crucial to maintain the airway so that continuous gas flow is maintained for exchange.

Airway management in critically ill patients differs significantly from induction of anesthesia and intubation. In this chapter we will discuss airway management as:

- Airway assessment
- Airway interventions
- Extubation
- Drugs for airway management.

AIRWAY ASSESSMENT

Airway assessment is done with regards to:

- Patency
- Protective reflexes
- Respiratory drive
- Ambient air.

Airway Patency

It describes clean and clear passage for air flow. If a person is talking coherently it means the airway is patent. The hallmark of airway obstruction is diminished or absent airflow in the presence of repeated inspiratory effort by the patient. Any sound during breathing signifies partial airway obstruction. While wheezing signifies lower respiratory tract obstruction;

Table 1: Causes of airway obstruction

Causes of abnormal airway patency
Obstruction: Secretions, blood, vomitus, foreign bodies, inhalation burn, edema, trauma
Anatomical: Short neck, congenital anamalies, obesity, ankylosing spondylitis
Neurological: Coma, trauma, etc.
Drugs: Opioid overdose, sedatives

loud sounds like stridor usually signify upper airway obstruction. The triple airway maneuver is used to relieve airway obstruction following which adjuncts such as oro or nasopharyngeal airway is used.

Protective Reflexes

These reflexes help to keep the airway open and to remove secretion. The main two reflexes are swallowing and cough reflexes.

Respiratory Drive and Ambient Air

Airway patency once ensured has to be followed by breathing and oxygen supply. Breathing is to be supported if respiratory efforts are inadequate. If patient is hypoxic (SpO_2 <90%) oxygen supplementation is needed.

AIRWAY INTERVENTIONS

These are life saving maneuver done to ensure emergency oxygenation in a patient with compromised airway. The person managing the airway should be at the head end of the patient and the patient is lying supine with head in neutral position. The person managing the airway should wear protective gears. A airway management trolley and crash cart should be available. Suction facility with 120 mm Hg pressure and oxygen source is mandatory

The airway trolley and crash cart should contain all the essential equipment and drugs (Table 2). A multi-parameter

Table 2: Equipment in emergency crash cart*

Airway trolley equipment
Suction: Yankauer tube and PVC suction catheters of different sizes
Nasogastric tube **Airways:** Nasopharyngeal and oropharyngeal
Bag mask ventilation with reservoir bag and O_2 tube
Direct laryngoscope with different blades
Cuffed endotracheal tube of different sizes with tie for fixation
Stillete and flexible Bougie
Laryngeal mask airway

(*all the equipments should be of different sizes)

monitor with ECG, SpO_2, end tidal CO_2 and NIBP measurement facility must be attached to the patient. If the patient is responsive please seek his cooperation and inform him before intervention, if needed use drugs as described later.

The airway intervention can be broadly classified into two:

1. Emergency unresponsive patient
2. Elective airway management.

Emergency Unresponsive Patients

Assess for airway patency as mentioned before. If the patient has patent airway and is unresponsive put the patient in *stable lateral position* and observe.

If the airway is not patent then stand on head end and do *head tilt and chin lift maneuver* to open the airway. In suspected cervical trauma patient head tilt is not recommended and only *jaw thrust* is to be done.

Once the airway is open, look for any secretions, blood etc obstructing the airway. Clean the airway under vision by suction using Yankauer suction.

To maintain the patency use appropriate size nasopharyngeal or oropharyngeal airway. Nasopharyngeal airway is used in persons with intact gag reflex and oropharyngeal is used in patients with absent gag.

After clearing the airway assess for breathing and if inadequate then start bag and mask ventilation. Use correct size mask with O_2 source. Use self-inflating bag (ÄMBU) to ventilate. Sellick maneuver (cricoid pressure) may be used to reduce the risk of aspiration especially in full stomach patients.

However for prolonged ventilation and transport of such patients to ICU definitive airway is indicated.

Securing definitive airway in emergency situation needs a lot of skill and experience. A quick assessment for difficult airway must be done before intervention. In case of anticipated difficulty use LMA (size 3 for female; size 4 for male) otherwise endotracheal intubation is the gold standard.

ELECTIVE AIRWAY MANAGEMENT

The planned securing of airway by endotracheal intubation is done in stable patients for mechanical ventilation.

Steps in Securing Airway Electively

1. Preoxygenate the patient with non rebreathing O_2 mask and attach ECG, pulse oximeter and BP monitor. If available keep end tidal CO_2 monitor ready.
2. Keep ready all the airway equipments, difficult airway gadgets and crash cart at the bedside. Secure an iv line for medication.
3. Do a quick assessment of the airway for anticipated difficulty. There are many ways to assess the airway one such is 'LEMON'

Table 3: Assessment for anticipated difficult airway—LEMON

L: Look for facial trauma or any abnormality
E: Evaluate 3-3-2 rule 3 finger interincisor gap 3 finger hyomental distance 2 finger thyrohyoid distance
M: Mallampati: score of airway Class 1 : Post-pharyngeal wall and tonsillar pillar visible on mouth opening Class 2 : Uvula visible Class 3 : Base of uvula and soft palate visible Class 4 : Soft palate not visible
O: Obstruction of airway
N: Neck movements restriction especially extension

where a quick anticipation of difficult airway can be made (Table 3).

Abnormality of any of the above might cause difficult visualization of airway by direct laryngoscopy and endotracheal intubation.

4. In ICU endotracheal intubation is a challenge and a proper planning is needed. Always expert help must be around. These patients are prone to hypoxemia with poor reserve and catastrophe may happen if not planned well.
5. In case of failed attempt of intubation modified difficult airway algorithm of ASA may be used (Fig. 1).
6. Unlike in OT failed intubation is poorly tolerated in ICU due to poor reserve and associated other abnormality. If failed then secure the airway with LMA or surgically (cricothyrotomy or emergency tracheostomy).

EXTUBATION

Extubation is done when the patient is fully awake and is expected to protect his airway. Anticipated to maintain airway and oxygenation spontaneously.

Always perform cuff leak test before extubation. It rules out cord edema and risk of stridor post-extubation. Similar to intubation extubation can be life threatening and same level of care and equipments needed. Various extubation criteria has been described of which rapid shallow breathing index (RSBI) is most well validated. RSBI is calculated by respiratory rate (per min) divided by tidal volume (in liters). A value less than 100–105 is considered appropriate for extubation.

Withhold feeds for two hours before and after extubation. Routine use of steroids and prokinetic drugs to facilitate gastric emptying is not recommended.

Inform the patient about extubation and seek their cooperation. Ask the patient to take a deep breath 'deflate the endotracheal tube, cuff and remove the ET tube at peak inspiration to minimize cord trauma. In COPD patients elective application of non invasive ventilation is a good practice. One

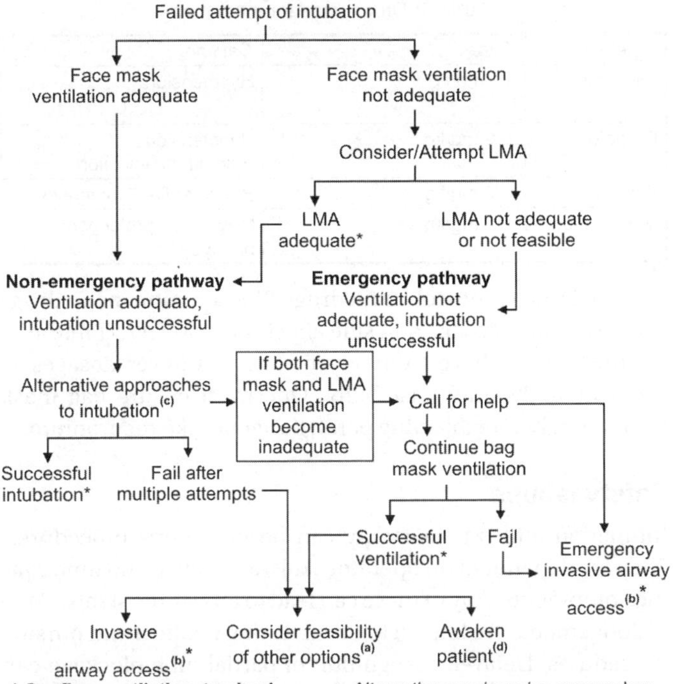

*** Confirm ventilation, tracheal intubation, or LMA placement with exhaled CO_2**

a. Other options include (but are not limited to): surgery utilizing face mask or LMA anesthesia, local anesthesia in filtration or regional nerve blockade. Pursuit of these options usually implies that mask ventilation will not be problematic. Therefore, these options may be of limited value it this step in the algorithm has been reached via the emergency pathway.

b. Invasive airway accoss includes surgical of parcutaneous tracheostomy or cricothyrotomy.

c. Alternative non-invasive approaches to difficulty intubation include (but are not limited to): use of different laryngoscope blades, LMA as an intubation conduit (with or without fiberoptic guidance), fiberoptic intubation, intubating stylet or tube changer, light wand, retrograde intubation, and blind oral or nasal intubation.

d. Consider re-preparation of the patient for awake intubation. or canceling surgery

e. Options for emergency non-invasive airway ventilation include (but are not limited to): rigid bronchoscope, esophageal tracheal combitube ventilation, or transtracheal jet ventilation.

Fig. 1: Modified Difficult airway algorithm for ICU (*Source:* American Society of Anesthesiology (ASA) from ASA algorithm of difficult airway).

must remember that upto 15% of patients get re-intubated within 48 hours of extubation.

Drugs in Airway Management

These drugs are:

- Sedative
- Analgesics
- Neuromuscular blocking agents.

All these drugs should be used cautiously in these patients as rapid administration can lead to hemodynamic abnormality. No standard recommendation is possible and every institution

Table 4: Drugs used for intubation

Agent	*Dose*	*Caution*
Midazolam	0.1 mg/kg	Hypotension
Propofol	1–2 mg/kg	Hypotension Pain during injection
Fentanyl	1–2 mg/kg	Bradycardia, hypotension
Rocuronium	1–2 mg/kg	May cause prolonged paralysis

have their own protocol about drugs. The common major drugs used with their dosage and side effects are shown in Table 4.

These drugs have to be given slowly in lower dosages to avoid hemodynamic instability. One must ensure bag mask ventilation before injecting paralytic agents like rocuronium.

Safety Issues

Intubation and tracheostomy can be hazardous procedures. They are dependent on operator skills, assistance and functioning equipments. Any of these can lead to airway incidents. Tube dislodgements are known to occur during medical and nursing procedures. Delayed recognition of partial tube blockage can have disastrous consequences. Given the many possibilities of airway incidents it is clear that all ICUs should have systems in place to address these issues.

3
CHAPTER

Oral Care

Prajakta Samir Hindlekar

ORAL CARE IN THE INTENSIVE CARE UNIT

The experience of a fresh, clean mouth following cleaning one's teeth is universal. This is an activity that most individuals undertake daily. Oral care for patients in the hospital's intensive care unit (ICU) is important. Lack of skill in performing oral assessment, inadequate evidence based guidelines on frequency of oral care are challenges faced by critical care nurses. This chapter will focus on of current trends in oral care in ICU followed by recommendations.

Oral care is a key component of nursing care in the ICU. Often it is considered primarily an intervention for patients' comfort, a characteristic that may reduce its priority and thus its frequency. Precise information about the frequency and type of oral care will guide the development of nursing interventions that may improve outcomes in these patients.

Study done by Ante Jordan and Ana Badovinac et al. in 2014 among total of 241 ICU nursing staff across 14 public hospitals in Croatia, revealed that most nurses provided oral care for patients in ICU's 2–3 times a day (65%). Gauze soaked with paraffin oil and rinsing the oral cavity with chlorhexidine were the most frequently performed tasks (74.7% and 58.1%, respectively). Lack of time (58.1%), inadequate staff (48.5%), supplies and equipment (44.4%) were the main barriers to provision of oral care.

INTUBATION, ARTIFICIAL VENTILATION AND ORAL COLONIZATION

Change in oropharyngeal colonization has been implicated in the pathogenesis of ventilator-associated pneumonia (VAP). Risk factors for VAP include the presence of an endotracheal tube and continuous ventilatory support. It is well established that presence of an endotracheal tube allows the direct entry of bacteria into the pulmonary tract, impairs the cough reflex, slows the action of the mucociliary escalator, and promotes excessive secretion of mucus. Additional risk factors include enteral nutrition therapy, lack of head end elevation and dental plaque.

Within 48 hours of hospital admission, the composition of the oropharyngeal flora of critically ill patients undergoes a change to predominantly gram-negative organisms. Dental plaque may serve as a reservoir for pathogens in patients with poor oral hygiene, and dental plaque of patients in the ICU is colonized by potential respiratory pathogens such as methicillin-resistant *Staphylococcus aureus* (MRSA) and *Pseudomonas aeruginosa*. This process of oral colonization usually precedes pulmonary colonization, which leads to VAP. Reducing the number of microorganisms in the mouth reduces the pool of organisms available for translocation to and colonization of the lung. Research indicates that vigorous oral hygiene is necessary to reduce oral colonization. Tooth brushing is effective in reducing the number of oral microorganisms, but tooth brushing, even though it is an independent nursing action, is not routinely performed in critically ill patients.

Unfortunately, although the importance of oral care in the ICU has been reported, there is limited research about the effects of oral care interventions in critically ill patients. Evidence-based protocols for oral care of critically patients are not available, and oral hygiene measures are generally directed toward patients' comfort rather than removal of microbes. The lack of published protocols for oral care in intubated patients has been noted in the clinical nursing literature. Definitive scientific studies relating oral care interventions to VAP have not been done. In a recent comprehensive research review of evidence-based practice related to strategies to prevent VAP, Hixson et al. noted that even though oral hygiene is considered standard nursing care. Hixson et al. called for studies evaluating the effectiveness of various methods of oral care.

ORAL ASSESSMENT

Despite the presence of the essential tools that can be used for oral assessment in ICUs, they are often not used. This may be due to a lack of time or knowledge on part of the bedside nurse as well as the lack of assistance for nurses in identifying particular problems such as candida or herpes simplex infections. Collaborative interactions with dental hygienists could improve the nurse's knowledge and skill related to oral care. A research-based protocol for oral care in the ICU setting is desirable.

ORAL CARE PRACTICES AND FREQUENCY

According to the nursing literature, toothbrushes are not the tools of choice for oral care by nurses. However, there is strong evidence to support the use of a toothbrush for the effective control of plaque and its associated complications; the toothbrush is recommended to be the tool of choice for mouth care. The most frequently used method involves the use of gauze soaked in an antiseptic solution, 1–4 times per day. Some solutions and types of equipment used by nurses for oral care are not optimal. Hydrogen peroxide and sodium bicarbonate effectively remove debris, but if not diluted carefully, may cause superficial burns. Foam swabs are effective for stimulation of mucosal tissues but are ineffective in removing plaque. Tooth brushing with fluoride toothpaste is advised for almost all patients.

The frequency of oral hygiene for intubated patients is an area of controversy. It is suggested that it should be done every 2–4 hours, depending on the patient's condition. More detailed research in this area is needed.

Challenges to Oral Care in Critical Care

- **Mechanical obstacles:** Mechanical obstructions challenge efficient and effective oral hygiene. The mouth of the ventilated intensive care patient is crowded with devices such as endotracheal and oral gastric tubes and occasionally a temperature probe. Tape or other device securing the endotracheal tube (ETT) in place presents a further obstacle when attempting to clean the patient's mouth.
- **Inadequate tools**
- **Perceptions of importance and patient discomfort by the nurse:** Maintaining patient safety and comfort also impact on decisions with regard to the frequency and type of mouth care administered by intensive care nurses. That is, some nurses have expressed the concerns related to oral care are dislodging the ETT, failing to remove all toothpaste and risk of aspiration of the mouth rinse used when providing oral hygiene (Kite and Pearson, 1995).
- **Patient perception and discomfort issues:** In addition to mechanical barriers, individual patient factors may also pose a challenge to the provision of mouth care. This may include a procedure such as mouth care which the patient may dread but is perceived by the nurse as being very basic and completely painless. In addition, due to the administration of sedatives and analgesics, almost all ICU patients experience some degree of confusion at some time during their stay in ICU (Rundshagen et al. 2002; Roberts et al. 2005). This altered perception of reality experienced by the patient may confound attempts by the nurse to thoroughly clean the patient's mouth and therefore result in a rudimentary swabbing of the patient's teeth and gums with only a cotton or foam swab stick. If the patient is in pain, there may be a reluctance to comply with the attempted practice of mouth care, once more resulting in inadequate care being provided.

- **Communication barriers:** Due to the possible confusion mentioned above and the presence of the ETT, ICU patients have a reduced capacity to communicate. This lack of ability to speak can often be the source of gross irritation and frustration for the patient which may also lead to lack of compliance with oral hygiene.

It is clearly evident from the review chapter on oral care in ICU that there is paramount need for research based recommendations on oral care in ICU. Nursing curriculum should emphasize on oral care during the clinical training. It is to be regarded as important hands on skill needing frequent ongoing training in the ICU.

FURTHER READING

1. Adams R. Qualified nurses lack adequate knowledge related to oral health, resulting in inadequate oral care of patients on medical wards. J Adv Nurs. 1996;24(3):552-60.
2. Berry AM, Davidson PM. Beyond comfort: Oral hygiene as a critical nursing activity in the intensive care unit. Intensive Crit Care Nurs. 2006; 22(6):318-28.
3. Chan EY, Hui-Ling Ng 1: Oral care practices among critical care nurses in Singapore: a questionnaire survey. Appl Nurs Res. 2012; 25(3):197-204.
4. Jones H, Newton J, Bower EJ. A survey of the oral care practices of intensive care nurses. Intensive Crit Care Nurs. 2004;20:69-76.
5. Jordan A, Badovinac A, et al. Factors influencing intensive care nurses' knowledge and attitudes regarding ventilator-associated pneumonia and oral care practice in intubated patients in Croatia. Am J Infect Control, 2014;42(10):1115-7.
6. O'Reilly M. Oral care of the critically ill: a review of the literature and guidelines for practice. Aust Crit Care. 2003;16(3):101-10.

4
CHAPTER

Eye Care

Prajakta Samir Hindlekar

Eye care is recognized as a basic nursing care procedure essential for critically ill patients to prevent complications such as eye infection or injury. Standards of care delivered in critical care units (CCU) cannot be complete without including eye care clinical practice guideline.

INTRODUCTION

Many critically ill patients have altered levels of consciousness which may impact on the protective mechanisms of the eye. When unprotected, the eye is at risk of injury, such as corneal dehydration, abrasion, perforation and infection. The reported incidence rates for corneal abrasion vary widely in the international health care literature; 3–60% intensive care patients are affected. The provision of fundamental eye care to this patient population is essential and particularly important in the first 2–7 days, when the peak incidence of iatrogenic eye injury occurs.

REVIEW ON SIGNIFICANCE OF PROTECTIVE PHYSIOLOGICAL MECHANISMS IN THE EYE

An important consideration to guiding assessment and management is to have thorough understanding of the normal physiological mechanisms that provide protection against eye injury and infection.

1. Eyelid closure and blinking provide a mechanical barrier to injury and prevent dehydration and the desiccation of the outer eye epithelium.
2. Conjunctiva, the thin protective layer of epithelium that forms a mucous membrane covering the anterior surface of the eye, protects the eye from mechanical injury and invasion from micro-organisms.
3. Tear formation is an important component of the outer eye defense mechanisms. Tears maintain a moist environment for the surface epithelium of the outer eye and form a smooth optical surface over the cornea. Tears lubricate the eyelids, wash away foreign material and cell debris, prevent adherence of organisms to the ocular surface, and transport

oxygen to the outer eye surface. In the event of injury or infection, leukocytes are transferred to the injured area in tear fluid. Additionally, proteins such as immunoglobulin, lysozyme and lactoferrin are found in tears and inhibit bacterial growth. The action of blinking facilitates the distribution of tears to the whole of the ocular surface.

ALTERED EYE PHYSIOLOGY IN CRITICALLY ILL PATIENTS

For the critically ill patient, normal protective mechanisms such as eyelid closure during sleep and an intact blink reflex may be altered because of the use of sedation and muscle relaxants or because of underlying medical conditions that alter the patient's level of consciousness. Sedation and the use of neuromuscular blocking agents affect the orbicular muscles of the eye and the eyelid may appear to be closed. However lagophthalmos (incomplete eyelid closure) may still occur, contributing to drying of the mucosal surface and desiccation of the epithelial tissues and may result in ulceration (exposure keratopathy). The resulting lesions can range from punctate epithelial erosions involving the exposed inferior third of the cornea to more extensive erosion or macro-epithelial defect. The disruption to the epithelial surface increases the risk of bacterial infection.

In addition to the alteration of normal eye protective mechanisms, the intensive care unit (ICU) environment also presents an environment rich in pathogens that may contribute to the increased exposure of the ocular surface to microorganisms.

For these reasons meticulous eye care is required to minimize the development of iatrogenic ophthalmologic complications, which, if not resolved, may result in serious visual impairment.

POTENTIAL EYE PROBLEMS FOR CRITICALLY ILL PATIENTS

1. Superficial keratopathy, which is a non-inflammatory disease of the cornea due to exposure and drying of the eye which can lead to ulceration, perforation and scarring, which though usually self-limiting, may cause permanent damage.
2. Superficial corneal abrasions which are common, due to eye exposure.
3. Keratitis which refers to any inflammation of the cornea, and in particular relates to infection. Bacterial or exposure keratitis is considered a dire complication associated with corneal exposure.
4. Inflammation of the conjunctiva, termed conjunctivitis, is also a risk and is caused by bacterial or viral infection, allergy or environmental factors.

In the ear of accreditation, corneal abrasions, conjunctival edema and infection have commonly been cited as adverse events.

INCIDENCE OF COMMON EYE PROBLEMS

Current literature suggests that the incidence of corneal abrasions ranged from 3.33% to 22% of the intensive care population. During a prospective analysis of 50 randomly selected intensive care patients, one study found corneal abrasions in 40% of patients. Another study suggested that up to 60% of ICU patients who receive sedation for longer than 48 hours may get corneal abrasions, and that the majority of these were detected in the first week of admission.

Existing Eye Care Practices

Eye care for intubated and ventilated patients receiving sedation or muscle relaxation varies greatly between intensive care units in terms of the method and frequency of eye care. Eye care has generally involved a regimen of cleaning the eyes every 2–4 hours with sterile water or normal saline and the installation of a lubricating liquid such as methylcellulose. Eye ointment is used where there is evidence of eye injury or the risk of injury is thought to be increased, for instance where conjunctival edema is present. Where there is evidence of conjunctival or corneal exposure, methods such as eye taping, padding, application of ointment, and application of polyethylene film are described, however, from the available evidence it is unclear, if any of these methods contribute to ocular surface protection separate from their contribution to eyelid closure. Because of the dearth of research about eye care in the critically ill patient population, it is also unclear which of these is most effective in maintaining eyelid closure.

Recommendations from various studies searched related to eye care in critical care unit are as follows:

Assessment Guidelines

1. Each patient is assessed for:
   - Risk factors of iatrogenic ophthalmologic complications
   - Ability to maintain eyelid closure and
   - Iatrogenic ophthalmologic complications.
2. Frequency of assessment: every 2–4 hours.

Eye Care Recommendations

1. Eye care should be part of the care provided to all people during their admission to intensive care units.
2. Ointments and drops are more effective at reducing the incidence of corneal abrasions than no eye instillations.

3. Polyethylene covers (Gladwrap) are more effective at reducing the incidence of corneal abrasions than ointments and drops.
4. Eyelid closure to be maintained if eyelid closure cannot be maintained passively; all patients who cannot achieve eyelid closure independently should receive eye care every 2 hours, i.e. cleaning with saline soaked gauze and the administration of an eye specific lubricant.
5. A timely referral is made for any suspected iatrogenic ophthalmologic complications.
6. Monitoring the rates of iatrogenic ophthalmologic complications. It is to be included as one of critical care quality indicators.

There is evidence that the eye care practice is given low priority, one need to have further studies to get in-depth information on recommendations for assessment, specific care and monitoring of ophthalmological complications together with best practice recommendations for prevention not included in previous eye care guidelines.

One needs to ensure dissemination and implementation of guidelines, which will improve eye care practices and morbidity for ICU patients. Inclusion of ophthalmological complications in quality of care performance indicators will have the dual effect of increasing awareness and highlighting areas for improvement in the practice of preventing potentially catastrophic ophthalmological complications. Early identification and prompt referral to ophthalmology experts has the potential to enhance patient outcomes.

FURTHER READING

1. de França CF, Fernandes AP. Evidence of interventions for the risk of dry eye in critically ill patients: An integrative review. Appl. Nurs. Res. 2016;29:14-17.
2. Marshall AP, Elliott R, Rolls K, Schacht S, Boyle M. Eyecare in the critically ill: clinical practice guideline. Aust. Cri. Care. 2008;21:97-109.
3. Rosenberg JB., Eisen LA. Eye care in the intensive care unit: narrative review and meta-analysis. Crit. Care Med. 2008;36(12); 3151-5.

5
CHAPTER

Pressure Sores

Prajakta Samir Hindlekar

PRESSURE ULCER

A pressure ulcer (PU) is localized injury to the skin and/or underlying tissue, usually over a bony prominence as a result of pressure or pressure in combination with shear and/or friction (NPUAP—National Pressure Ulcer Advisory Panel 2009). The most common site for pressure ulcers is the sacrum, with heels being second.

Preventing pressure ulcers is an important nursing concern for hospitalized patients. Intensive care unit (ICU) patients are at higher risk for pressure ulcer development due to comorbidities and life-saving treatment modalities in this environment. The incidence of pressure ulcer ranges from 8.8 to 23%.

Although several nursing interventions have been advocated in the literature, there is a paucity of research on what constitutes the most effective nursing intervention.

Pressures Ulcers are Staged from I to IV

- Stage I is intact skin with non-blanchable redness of a localized area
- Stage II is partial thickness loss of dermis presenting as a shallow open ulcer with a red or pink wound bed, without slough
- Stage III is full thickness tissue loss where subcutaneous fat may be visible but bone, tendon or muscles are not exposed
- Stage IV is full thickness tissue loss with exposed bone, tendon or muscle (NPUAP and EPUAP—European Pressure Advisory Panel, 2009).

Two additional stages are recognized by the NPUAP and are unstageable which is full thickness tissue loss in which actual depth of the ulcer is completely obscured by slough and suspected deep tissue injury which is of unknown depth with a purple or maroon localized area of discolored intact skin or blood-filled blister due to damage of underlying soft tissue from pressure and/or shear.

Hospital-acquired Pressure Ulcer

A hospital-acquired pressure ulcer (HAPU) is defined as any ulcer noted 24 or more hours after hospital admission.

Because pressure ulcer staging is dependent on visible skin characteristics, a great potential for misclassifying pressure-related injury exists.

Deep Tissue Injury

Deep tissue injury (DTI) can remain undetected for days or weeks before a purple discoloration of the skin appears. In patients with very dark skin, a DTI may not be visible at all, especially in the area of the gluteal fold where skin color is darker. Thus, often a patient may be in the hospital for several days and develop an HAPU even though it was most likely present underneath on admission (Gefen, Farid, and Shaywitz, 2013). Studies suggest that deep tissue is more susceptible than superficial tissue to injury caused by externally applied pressure; clinically superficial skin injuries induced by pressure tend to be associated with deep tissue damage; and superficial injuries appear to be caused by factors other than pressure. The cause and development of a DTI is multifactorial with recent evidence that biomechanical forces, morphological changes and inflammation together with ischemia and aging, play a role in pressure ulcer pathogenesis (Berlowitz and Brienza, 2007; Stojadinovic et al. 2013).

In the developed counties, insurance companies consider pressure sores reasonably preventable and have halted reimbursement for the treatment of hospital-acquired pressure ulcers (HAPUs) stages II to IV, unless they were determined to have been present at admission or within 2 days after admission. However, clinicians argue that some pressure ulcers are unavoidable and will occur even when all the necessary interventions are implemented. Examples of these conditions are hemodynamic instability requiring pharmacologic or mechanical support which diminish perfusion, severe protein-energy malnutrition which alters tissue tolerance, or skin breakdown in terminally ill individuals. In addition, because pressure ulcers are preventable in most situations, they have resulted in litigation, with settlements often favoring patients.

Based on these facts, most hospitals in developed countries have established protocols and interventions for preventing or lessening the severity of pressure ulcers. Despite a variety of prevention and treatment modalities for pressure ulcers there is limited consensus on the best interventions, with a paucity of randomized clinical trials (RCTs) to provide conclusive clinical practice guidelines. Extensive interventions for the prevention of pressure ulcers in the past 5 to 10 years in most developed countries has resulted in significant decrease in HAPUs. However similar decreases in prevalence rates including patients with pressure ulcers at the time of hospital admission have not been achieved.

The following interventions have been used to prevent pressure ulcers to date.

1. Patient repositioning: Being basic tenet of nursing care, there is limited empirical evidence of the effect of positioning on the prevention of pressure ulcers.
2. Nutrition and vitamins
3. Support surfaces: The use of special beds, mattresses, sheets and overlays designed to redistribute pressure, have been widely used to prevent pressure sores since the mid-1980s. Several RCTs found that using special mattresses or sheets significantly reduce the incidence of pressure ulcers.
4. Skin care: In the presence of pressure and shear forces both excess moisture and dryness can exacerbate skin breakdown, making a patient more susceptible to a pressure ulcers. A recent systematic review (Clark et al., 2014) found only one high-quality randomized controlled trial (RCT). Nevertheless, based on descriptive and cohort studies, they concluded that dressings such as hydrocellular, hydrocolloid or silicone foam dressings as part of pressure ulcer prevention may help reduce pressure ulcer incidence associated with medical devices and in immobile ICU patients.
5. Risk assessment: Many hospitals around the world have adopted risk assessment tools to evaluate patients at risk for developing pressure ulcers. A recent meta-analysis of 57 studies using different risk assessment scales found that the Braden, Norton, EMINA (mEntal state, Mobility, Incontinence, Nutrition, Activity), Waterlow, and Cubbin-Jackson scales showed the highest predictive capacity while a Cochrane review found only 2 RCTs and concluded that there is no reliable evidence to suggest that the use of structured, systematic pressure ulcer risk assessment tools reduces the incidence of pressure ulcers. The three

Table 1: Braden scale

Score	*Sensory Perception*	*Moisture*	*Activity Confined to bed*	*Mobility*	*Nutrition*	*Friction*
1	Completely limited	Very moist	Confined to bed	Completely immobile	Very poor	Maximum assistance
2	Very limited	Occasionally	Confined to chair	Very limited	Probably inadequate	Minimum assistance
3	Slightly limited	Rarely	Occasionally walks	Slightly change of position	Adequate	Maintains good position
4	No impairment	Never	No limitation	No limitation	Excellent	

Minimum risk = 16, Moderate risk = 13–14, Increased risk = 12 or less most widely used instruments are the Braden, the Norton and the Waterlow scales with the Braden scale having the highest pooled predictive capacity followed by the Norton scale and the Waterlow scale.

6. Multiple interventions: More benefits of multi-pronged interventions in reducing pressure sores in intensive care units have been documented.

INTACT: The Bundle Approach for the Prevention of Hapus

I: Incontinence

- Clean skin regularly and keep it dry
- Offer toileting regularly
- Use fecal/urinary collection systems
- Use barrier films/creams over perineal area
- Assess and change diapers frequently.

N: Nutrition

- Consult dietitian and ensure optimal nutritional intake
- Follow up any recent weight loss
- Maintain adequate hydration unless contraindicated.

T: Turning

- Turn patient every 2 hours and when needed while in bed
- Shift patient's weight when in chair every:
  - One hour when patient needs assistance
  - Fifteen minutes when patient can move freely.
- Relieve pressure points over bony prominences
- Do not drag patient
- Elevate head of bed, hands, and heels.

A: Assessment

- Assess patient's skin upon admission and every shift
- Assess risk for impaired skin integrity
- Assess bed sheets for wrinkles and soiling
- Avoid hypothermia
- Avoid positioning patient on existing pressure ulcer and over tubes.

C: Consultation

- Consult physical therapist.

Charting

- Chart skin and risk assessment findings, prevention interventions, and education.

T: Teaching

- Teach patient/family to:
  - Inspect susceptible body prominences
  - Perform appropriate prevention measures
  - Avoid aggressive massaging and rubbing over bony prominences.

The fact that HAPUs are best predicted by skin care management and lower Braden scores, nurses should ensure that these cost effective measures are part of routine care of patients in ICU's. There are multifaceted interventions which include: administrative support with active involvement of trained nursing staff with safe ratios at the patient care level, developing a bundle of care which is infused into routine care practice, and accurate documentation. However, most of these interventions are based on clinical judgment and consensus rather than on sound research.

Monitoring trends of pressure ulcer rates and analysis should guide institutional efforts to improve incidence of pressure ulcers. Tracking weekly pressure sore prevalence and having it available to the care givers is proven to be an innovative strategy to prevent HAPU's in ICU's. Customized initiatives will cater to the needs of both patients and professionals in each ICU. It is also important that successful initiatives be maintained and sustained to ensure that the changes are embedded into practice.

FURTHER READING

1. Ballard N, McCombs A, Deboor S, Strachan J, Johnson M, Smith MJ, et al. How our ICU decreased the rate of hospital-acquired pressure ulcers. J Nurs Care Qual. 2008;23(1):92-6.
2. Chou R, Dana T, Bougatsos C, Blazina I, Starmer AJ, Reitel K, et al. Pressure ulcer risk assessment and prevention: a systematic comparative effectiveness review. Ann Intern Med. 2013;159(1):28-38.
3. Dirksen, Shannon Ruff, Lewis, Sharon L, Heitkemper, Margaret McLean, et al. Companion to Medical Surgical Nursing. 9th edition: Mosby, 2014.
4. Krupp AE, Monfre J. Pressure ulcers in the ICU patient: an update on prevention and treatment. Curr Infect Dis Rep. 2015;17(3):468.
5. Mallah Z, Nassar N, Kurdahi Badr L. The Effectiveness of a pressure ulcer intervention program on the prevalence of hospital acquired pressure ulcers: Controlled before and after study. Appl Nurs Res. 2015;28(2):106-13.
6. McInnes E, Jammali-Blas A, Bell-Syer SE, Dumville JC, Cullum N. Support surfaces for pressure ulcer prevention. Cochrance Database Syst Rev. 2011;(4):CD001735.
7. Pieper B. Acute and Chronic Wounds: 5th(edn), Elsevier. 2016; 124-39.

6 CHAPTER

Physiotherapy in Intensive Care Unit

Vasudha Sethi

INTRODUCTION

Physiotherapists are an integral part of the intensive care unit (ICU) team. They are uniquely qualified with skills and expertise to work with the assessment and management of respiratory complications, ICU acquired weakness and related conditions.

Chest physical therapy is often necessary due to retained secretions following intubation and immobility.

- To improve respiratory efficiency
- Promote expansion of lungs
- Strengthen respiratory muscles
- Eliminate secretions from lungs.

INDICATIONS FOR CHEST PHYSIOTHERAPY

Acute Conditions

- Copious secretions
- Acute respiratory failure with retained secretions
- Acute lobar atelectasis.

Chronic Conditions

- Cystic fibrosis
- Bronchiectasis
- Chronic bronchitis
- Pneumonia
- Restrictive pulmonary disease.

Retention of Secretions may occur due to

- Recumbancy
- Post-surgery
- Prolonged mechanical ventilation
- Chronic pulmonary diseases
- Neurological injury
- Infusion of analgesics and sedatives.

Contraindication

- Undrained pneumothorax
- Raised intracranial pressure (ICP)

TECHNIQUES USED FOR CHEST PHYSIOTHERAPY

Bronchial Hygiene and Methods to Increase Lung Volumes

1. Deep breathing exercises
2. Incentive spirometry
3. Forced expiratory techniques
   - Tracheal stimulation
   - Huffing and coughing.

Postural Drainage

Mobilizing secretions so that the secretions move to central airways from where they can be suctioned. This can be done by placing patients in various positions so gravity assists the drainage process.

Techniques used with postural drainage percussion, vibration and shaking—drumming and shaking action on the chest wall to mobilize secretions voluntary or stimulated coughing.

Postural drainage is indicated in diseases which cause increase in production of mucus, such as chronic bronchitis, cystic fibrosis. It is also done in postoperative patients especially those who have undergone thoracic surgery.

Contraindications to postural drainage include:

1. Osteoporosis or rib fracture
2. Severe hemoptysis
3. Pulmonary edema
4. Pulmonary embolus
5. Asthma or bronchospasm
6. Pneumothorax
7. Hemodynamic instability including arrhythmias
8. Congestive cardiac failure
9. Neurosurgical patients with raised ICP
10. Ocular surgery.

HYPERINFLATION

This process involves hyperinflating to above 50% of the ventilator delivered tidal volume, aiming to expand collapsed alveoli and mobilize secretions. A recommended technique is slow inspiration, 1–2 seconds plateu phase, and then a rapid release of the bag to simulate a huff and mobilize secretions. Preoxygenation may be needed as PEEP may be lost and delivered tidal volume may be inadequate. Cardiac output often falls with variable blood pressure and heart rate responses. Sedation may blunt hemodynamic response. Full deflation avoids air trapping. This is followed by suction. A cough reflex may be stimulated to mobilize secretions further. Tenacious secretions can be loosened by instillation of 2–5 mL of normal saline.

COMPLICATIONS

- Hypoxemia: from suction, loss of PEEP, etc.
- Hemodynamic disturbance (may be related high tidal volume, airway pressure, hypoxemia, agitation, tracheal stimulation)
- Direct trauma from suctioning
- Barotrauma, including pneumothorax.

EARLY MOBILIZATION

The National Institute for Health and Care Excellence (NICE), the European Respiratory Society and the European Society of Intensive Care Medicine recommend early assessment and management of physical morbidity (including mobilization and muscle training) delivered by physiotherapists and other health professionals. They also recommend that the physiotherapist should be responsible for implementing mobilization plans and exercise prescription in conjunction with other team members.

Early mobilization of mechanically ventilated patients is safe, well-tolerated and has shown to result in early weaning, and lesser incidence of delirium.

In view of the new evidence demonstrating the effectiveness of physiotherapy interventions aimed at early mobilization, ICU physiotherapists should give priority to these interventions. However to be successful, implementation of early mobilization relies on an ICU culture that considers mobilization an essential part of multidisciplinary care.

FURTHER READING

1. Gosselink R, Bott J, Johnson M, et al. Physiotherapy for adult patients with critical illness: recommendations of the European Respiratory Society and European Society of Intensive Care Medicine Task Force on Physiotherapy for Critically Ill Patients. Intensive Care Medicine. 2008;34(7):1188-99.
2. National Institute for Health and Clinical Excellence. Rehabilitation after critical illness, CG83. London: National Institute for Health and Clinical Excellence; 2009.

7 CHAPTER

Fast Hugs Bid

Sanjay MV, Raymond D Savio

One of the effective means of delivering optimal care to patients in the intensive care unit (ICU) is by following a *bundle* approach, e.g. ventilator-associated pneumonia (VAP) bundle, catheter-related bloodstream infections (CRBSI) bundle, etc. One such very effective bundle is the FAST HUG. The idea was originally conceived and published in 2005 by Vincent JL. It has now evolved to include more components and therefore becomes FAST HUGS BID.

FAST HUG is the acronym for the following components:

- **F**eeding
- **A**nalgesia
- **S**edation
- **T**hromboprophylaxis
- **H**ead end elevation
- **U**lcer prophylaxis
- **G**lycemic control.

The components that have been later included are:

- **S**pontaneous breathing trial
- **B**owel care
- **I**ndwelling catheter removal
- **D**e-escalation of antibiotics.

FEEDING

Critical ill are generally hypercatabolic and becomes malnourished rapidly. This in turn leads to impaired wound healing, increased susceptibility to infection, organ dysfunctions, loss of lean body mass and adverse outcomes. Feeding is one of the most important components of the bundle to improve the outcome of the patient. Nutrition can thus be regarded a "therapy" and not just supplementation in the critically ill. Attempts should be made initiate feeding in patients as soon as possible.

Simple Check List Before Initiation

1. Assess all patients for their nutritional status on admission, or atleast within 24–48 hours of admission. Subjective global assessment (SGA), nutrition risk in criticall ill

(NUTRIC) score, nutrition risk screening (NRS) 2002 are the commonly used scores for nutritional risk assessment. A score of >3 for NRS 2002 or >5 for nutric suggests high-nutritional risk. Also consider patients' comorbidities, availability of GI tract, risk of aspiration before starting feeds.

2. Oral feeding is preferred. If the clinical condition is unfavorable, enteral feeding with tube gastric feeds or jejunal feeds is the next choice. This helps in maintaing the gut integrity, reduces gut translocation, reduces the incidence of infections and organ dysfunctions.
3. Gastric tolerance to feeds should be evaluated regularly. Feeds should not be delayed or withheld for mere absence of bowel sounds or high gastric residual volume (GRV). Looking for possible causes of altered gut motility, like drugs, metabolic, endocrine and electrolyte disturbances and correcting them helps in achieving the targets. Promotility drugs like metoclopramide and erythromycin can be considered if there are no overt signs of obstruction.
4. Keep the head end elevated to 30 degrees to avoid aspiration.
5. Calories are to be provided at 25 kcal/kg/day using carbohydrates (60–70%) and fats (30–40%). Proteins are to be provided at 1.2–2 g/kg/day and should not be calculated in the calorie intake. Weight is adjusted to baseline weight or lean body weight for the purpose of calculations. Feeds are as a fraction of the calculated calorie requirement on day 1 and can be increased over next 48–72 hours to reach the targets by the end of one week. Volume of the feeds should be adjusted according to the fluid balance of the previous 24 hours.
6. There is evidence that continuous feeds with well-maintained feeding bags or pumps improve tolerance to enteral feeds. Regular checking for gastric residual volume (GRV) is not mandatory. It can be done as and when required or based on institutional protocol. A GRV > 500 mL should prompt evaluation for GI intolerance.
7. Routine use of immunonutrition, antioxidants, arginine are not advised. They may be recommended in specific patient populations such as traumatic brain injury (TBI), burns and postsurgical settings.
8. Nutritional assessment should be done regularly (at least once every week) to assess the changing needs and therefore delivery.
9. Parenteral nutrition (PN) is to be considered in patients with high nutritional risk who are not able to achieve even 60% of the calorie and protein targets by 7–10 days. Either exclusive parenteral nutrition or combined (with enteral nutrition) can be considered. Various formulations are available and the product has to be selected according to the needs of the patient. PN should be delivered following

'strict aspetic precautions' through a dedicated central or peripheral (in the case of Peripheral PN) line. Special attention should be paid for a adequate glycemic control and electrolyte homeostasis.

10. Having an institutional protocol, training the staff and having dedicated dietary departments helps in better delivery of nutritional therapy.

ANALGESIA, SEDATION

Pain, agitation and delirium are unpleasant and very common. It could be detrimental in both short- and long-term. Acutely, it can cause exaggerated and uncontrolled neurohumoral response which leads to increased catabolism, impaired healing, accidental removal of tubes and lines, delayed extubations due to increased work of breathing/ventilatory asynchrony, adverse cardiac events, increased length of stay (LOS) in ICU and hospital, etc. Long-term adverse outcomes includes psychological trauma, posttraumatic stress disorder (PTSD), chronic pain, etc.

Optimal analgesia and sedation therefore plays a pivotal role in preventing and treating this unpleasant outcomes. Other therapies include antidelirium medication and nonpharmacological preventive strategies.

Analgesia can be pharmacological or nonpharmacological. It can preemptive or therapeutic and can be regional or systemic analgesia. Analgesic drugs can be divided into opioids and nonopioids. Multimodal analgesia with minimum possible interventions to keep the patient plays an important role in improving outcomes. Having *pain scales* to measure pain and titrate analgesia prevents both overtreating and undertreating the patient. *VAS* scale for neurologically intact patient and behavioral pain scales for others are the commonly used ones.

Selection of Drugs

Simple rule of thumb is to select drugs to provide effective analgesia with minimum possible or no side effects. *WHO pain ladder* protocol is simple and effective bedside tool that can be made use of.

Opiods

Fentanyl, Morphine, Tramadol, are the commonly used opioids in ICU. Drugs with high potency, short time for onset and short duration of action, with minimal effects of cardiorespiratory depression are preferred. Fentanyl fares better over other drugs for the above reasons. It can be given as intermittent boluses or infusions. Remifentanil is a very good choice for continuous infusions due its very rapid onset and very short duration of action. Itching, Ileus, drowsiness, and cardiorespiratory depression are the major side effects of opioids.

Non-opioids

Acetaminophen, other nonsteroidal anti-inflammatory drugs (NSAIDS) and NSAIDS are considered in this context. Common NSAIDS include diclofenac, ibuprofen and the newer COX-2 inhibitors. However, the NSAIDS are often avoided in an ICU setting owing to their significant adverse effect profile which includes nephrotoxicity, risk of GI bleed and inhibition of platelet function. Non-NSAIDS include ketamine and centrally acting alpha receptor agonists, e.g. clonidine and dexmedetomidine. Dexmedetomidine is especially gaining enormous popularity in ICU due ease of use and the fact that it allows for awake sedation coupled with analgesia. Bradycardia and hypotension may occur with bolus dosing.

Regional techniques like epidural nerve blocks, plexus blocks, peripheral nerve blocks, local infiltration of local anesthetics can be made use in a subset of postsurgical, trauma and malignancy-related patients.

THROMBOPROPHYLAXIS

Venous thromboembolism is a spectrum of disease, comprising of deep vein thrombosis (DVT) and pulmonary embolism (PE). The true incidence is much higher than what is quoted because of the nonspecific clinical findings. Many cases go either undiagnosed or unreported. Approximately 20–30% of the critically-ill patients experience DVT and most of them occur during the first 2 weeks of admission.

The VIRCHOW'S triad comprises of three crucial mechanisms, namely—*stasis, vascular endothelial injury and hypercoagulability*. When one or more of these are present, it predisposes to the development of DVT. The following are the risk factors for DVT under each mechanism.

Stasis

Atrial fibrillation, cardiac failure, prolonged immobility, venous insufficiency, venous obstruction.

Vascular Endothelial Injury

Trauma, surgery (major lower limb orthopedic surgery, lower abdominal, major surgeries), intravasular catheters, chemical irritation.

Hypercoagulation

Trauma, sepsis, malignany, systemic inflammatory response syndrome (SIRS), pregnancy, hormone replacement therapy (HRT), hereditary and acquired thrombophilias, nephrotic syndrome.

The risk for developing DVT–PE increases with the number of risk factors.

Several risk assessment systems are currently available. *Padua prediction score, improve risk assessment tool and the Revised Geneva score* are among the commonly used.

Thromboprophylaxis

The strategies adapted for the prevention of DVT can be classified as:

1. Primary prophylaxis—Strategies adapted to prevent DVT. This can be mechanical or chemical methods.
2. Secondary prophylaxis—Strategies adapted for early detection and treatment of subclinical venous thrombosis by screening with objective tests that are sensitive for the presence of DVT.

Primary prophylaxis is the best and effective way ahead and secondary prophylaxis is reserved for those in which primary prophylaxis is contraindicated or ineffective.

Mechanical Devices

These work by preventing venous stasis and have been proven to be better than no prophylaxis in high-risk patients. They are however less effective than chemical prophylaxis. The following are the methods for mechanical thromboprophylaxis.

1. Intermittent/sequential pneumatic compression devices.
2. Graded compression stockings.
3. Venous foot pumps.
4. Early mobilization.

These methods are chosen when there is a high risk for bleeding and where chemical prophylaxis cannot be used. In such cases, early transition to chemical prophylaxis is advised. In addition factors such as, chances of skin peeling, non-compliance due to patient discomfort and frequent removal make them less desirable. All attempts must be made for early mobilization if there are no contraindications.

Chemical Prophylaxis

Unfractionated Heparin (UFH)

Indirect thrombin inhibitor, acts by combining with anti-thrombin III and factor X. It is given at 5000 IU subcutaneous, twice daily. Complications include bleeding, heparin-induced thrombocytopenia (HIT) and osteoporosis. An eight hourly dosing can also be considered in high-risk subjects. It is safe for use in renal failure and pregnancy.

Low Molecular Weight Heparin (LMWH)

For example, enoxaparin, dalteparin act by anti-factor Xa activity. They have greater bioavailability and longer half life allowing single daily dose. They are proven to be more effective than UFH in preventing DVT in special high-risk situations such as post-orthopedic procedures. They are also better than UFH in terms of HIT, osteoporosis and do not need for laboratory monitoring.

- Enoxaparin—Dose 30 mg SC every 12 hours or 40 mg SC OD.
- Dalteparin—Dose 5000 IU SC daily. Postoperative dosing to be started after 12–24 hours.

Dose modifications are to be done in obesity and in renal failure. With Crcl <30 mL/minute.

Fondaparinux

This is a highly sulfated pentasaccharide and an indirect factor Xa inhibitor. The usual adult dose for thromboprophylaxis is 2.5 mg SC once daily (for body weight >50 kg). The advantages are a 100% bioavailability and a half life of 17 hours.

Newer Agents

Dabigatran, rivaroxaban, apixaban are newer agents that are slowly gaining popularity for certain specific indications.

Combining chemical and mechanical prophylaxis can also be considered in very high-risk instances for DVT.

HEAD END ELEVATION

Head end elevation in ICU is one of the most debated topics. The concept of head of bed (HOB) elevation was introduced to prevent the incidence of aspiration and the development of pneumonias. But the major setback of this is that it increases the chances of pressure ulcers in the sacral area in high-risk patients. So the questions about how much elevation and who all to receive HOB elevation is not completely answered.

Aspiration can happen with either oropharyngeal secretions or gastric contents or both. Neurological status (wakefullness), ability to maintain cough reflex, feeds and GI motility can all play a role in the incidence of aspiration. The response depends on the quantity, duration and type of aspirate. Symptoms can vary from being asymptomatic, to a chemical pneumonitis or to a full blown infective pneumonia. Most of earlier studies maintained HOB elevation at 45 degrees. They studied the effect of the same on incidence of aspiration and pneumonia. It proved to be beneficial in preventing aspiration but increased the incidence of pressure sores in the most dependant area, i.e. sacrum. Other limitations of greater HOB elevation are, limitation in turning the patient sideways, uncomfortable posture for sleeping. Head elevation cannot be applied in hemodynamically unstable, spine and pelvic fracture patients. Simple bedside practice is:

1. If no contraindications exist, HOB elevation of 45 degrees is to be offered to those at high risk for aspiration. Lesser degree can be considered (30 degrees) in those with a lower risk of aspiration.

2. Regular check is to be documented for pressure sores. Anti-pressure sore measures like maintaining good nutrition, perfusion, moisturization, reducing friction and early mobilization have to be strictly implemented.

ULCER PROPHYLAXIS

Stress-related ulceration of the upper gastrointestinal tract is known to be associated with critical illness. Clinical manifestations vary from asymptomatic lesions to significant GI bleeding. The incidence is quoted at 4% in critically-ill patients. Risk factors include:

- Shock
- Sepsis
- Hepatic failure
- Renal failure
- Major trauma including head injury, spinal cord injury
- Burns >35% of BSA
- Organ transplantation
- History of prior GI bleed.

Generally all patients in the ICU are candidates for stress ulcer prophylaxis unless there is contraindication to it.

Therapeutic Options

- Nutrition therapy
- Optimal hemodynamics
- H_2 receptor antagonists (H_2RA), e.g. ranitidine
- Proton pump inhibitors (PPIs), e.g. esomeprazole, pantoprazole, rabeprazole, etc.
- Sucralfate-mucosal protective agent
- Antacids (not a viable option as labor-intensive dosing regimes and side-effects).

High-risk populations benifit from PPIs compared to H_2RA in reducing clinically significant and overt GI bleed, but no mortality benefit has been observed. Studies have shown H_2RA to be better compared to sucralfate or antacids in preventing GI bleed in critically ill. Overall, none of the drugs have shown a mortality benefit.

Complications of Therapy

Proton Pump Inhibitors

- Interstitial nephritis
- *Clostridium difficile* enterocolitis
- Pneumonia (HAP and CAP)
- GI upset and headaches
- Long-term use associated with fractures, hypomagnesemia, hypocalcemia.

H_2 Blockers

- CNS side-effects

- Tolerance after 72 hours
- Drug allergy and drug interactions
- Pneumonia.

Simple Protocol

- Start enteral feeds as soon as feasible
- Risk stratify the patient based on risk factors
- Start on PPI for high risk patients or H_2RA for low to moderate risk patients
- If enteral feeding is feasible oral PPI to be preferred over IV
- If enteral feeding is not possible, IV PPI or H_2RA can be used depending on risk assessment
- Prompt de-escalation or stopping of the drugs is to be done when the risk is reduced
- Daily assessment and review is to be done to look for possible adverse effects.

GLYCEMIC CONTROL

Hyperglycemia in ICU is considered significant if blood glucose is >200 mg/dL. Hypoglycemia is severe when blood glucose <40–50 mg/dL and moderate when <70 mg/dL.

Abnormalities in blood sugar levels occur very frequently among the critically ill. Both are detrimental to patient outcomes. Depletion of glycogen stores, underfeeding, hypoglycemic agents and increased demand during stress contribute to the development of impaired glucose tolerance. Pre-existing diabetes mellitus, drugs (e.g. steroids), additional dextrose load can all contribute to hyperglycemias in the critically ill.

Various modalities are available for checking blood glucose. It can be measured in arterial, venous or capillary blood. Serum glucose measured from arterial blood sample in a laboratory is the most reliable but not always possible due to logistical reasons. Bedside estimation is commonly used in all due to its ease despite various limitations.

Normal blood glucose ranges from 80–110 mg/dL but during stress, hormonal changes induce a relative deficiency of insulin or insulin resistance, leading to hyperglycemic states. Hyperglycemia has been associated with increased incidence of infections, glycosuria, volume depletion, increased incidence of renal failure and ICU-acquired weakness. it also has proven to increase mortality among critially ill. Therefore great emphasis has to be given for preventing and treating hyperglycemias in critically ill.

Hypoglycemia is also quite common in ICU. The symptoms include dizziness, lightheadedness, blurring of vision, tiredness, sweating, etc. A large number of critically-ill patients will not be able to communicate leading to many instances of undetected and under-diagnosed hypoglycemia. Early recognition, glucose administration and correcting the underlying cause will prevent the complications associated with hypoglycemia. Studies have shown that maintaining tight glycemic control (70–110 mg/dL) have resulted in greater incidence of hypoglycemia and increased mortality. The present recommended goal is to maintain blood glucose between 140–180 mg/dL in the critically ill.

Short-acting IV insulin is the drug of choice for infusions during initial phase. Once the disease severity is reduced and the glycemic control is better one can switch to subcutaneous route. Long-acting insulins and oral hypoglycemic agents are best avoided in the critically-ill patient. Hypokalemia is a common occurrence with insulin infusions and care should be taken in providing potassium supplements.

SPONTANEOUS AWAKENING AND BREATHING TRIAL

The problems associated with undue and prolonged sedation of patients receiving mechanical ventilation have already been discussed and one of the more significant problems happen to be prolonged ventilation and its attendant morbidity. Several studies have proven the use of a Daily Sedation Interruption (DSI) also referred to as sedation holiday in early weaning. Likewise, a daily Spontaneous Breathing Trial (SBT) wherever appropriate, significantly cuts down on the number of ventilator and ICU days. Therefore combining a DSI with an SBT will be a more effective strategy towards early liberation of patients from MV.

BOWEL CARE

Both, diarrhea (defined as-2–3 liquid stools per day or >250 g of liquid stool per day) and constipation (defined as absence of evacuation of bowel contents for more than 3 consecutive days) are common in ICU. Etiology and consequences are many. This too contributes to ICU outcomes. Therefore daily careful monitoring for the frequency, quantity, consistency of the stools in ICU patients is important.

Diarrhea can be classified as infective and noninfective. Most commonly, it is noninfective in etiology resulting from feed intolerance, oral medications like laxatives, potassium chloride (KCl) syrup, oral phosphorous supplements, etc. Infective causes include *Clostridium difficile* or antibiotic-associated diarrhea. Diarrhea can also be classified as secretory and osmotic in nature. Osmotic diarrheas is of noninfective etiology whereas secretory diarrheas arise from infective etiologies. The test used to differentiate between the two is a stool osmolar gap. It is the difference between measured and calculated stool osmolality. If the difference is more than 100, it is suggestive of osmotic diarrhea. Feeds need not be stopped in the event of osmotic diarrhea, instead addition of soluble fibers and semielemental feeds can be considered. Signs like abdominal pain and tenderness, fever, leukocytosis, mucus and blood in stools favor the diagnosis of infective etiologies. Work-up for *Clostridium difficile* should be promptly undertaken in the presence of high-risk factors. Problems secondary to diarrhea of any etiology include alterations in fluid and electrolyte balance and loss of skin integrity and these have to be carefully attended.

Similarly, constipation is also very common in ICUs. Most common causes include opioids, dyselectrolytemias (hypokalemia), ileus, rarely *C. difficile* infection and intestinal obstruction. Evaluation involves a thorough abdominal examination assisted with laboratory and radiological tests where warranted. Surgical causes such as obstruction have to be promptly ruled out. Medical management includes treating metabolic causes like hypokalemia, hyperglycemias, withholding opioids/naloxone, etc. Laxatives and enemas can be considered where appropriate.

INDWELLING CATHETER REMOVAL

Catheters are commonly used in critically-ill patients. They are used for diagnostic, monitoring as well as therapeutic purposes. Commonly used ones are vascular catheters like central venous catheter, dialysis catheters, arterial catheters. Others include Foley's catheter, intercostals drains (ICD), surgical drains, lumbar drains, endotracheal tube, feeding tube, etc. Presence of catheters predispose to line related infections. They also creates some discomfort to the patients. Vascular catheters may also predispose to the development of thrombophlebitis and thromboembolism. Though all these lines are essential part of critical care, they come with a price. Therefore daily evaluation has to be made regarding the continued need for these lines and when no longer needed, they should be promptly removed.

DE-ESCALATION OF ANTIBIOTICS

Antimicrobial therapy is a very common and frequent therapeutic strategy in critical care. Since antibiotic resistance is on the rise and leads to poor clinical outcomes, it is the responsibility of every health care member to prevent their excessive use. Many protocols are in place to promote optimal use of antibiotics including prompt de-escalation when feasible. Reducing the use of antimicrobial agents also helps in reducing unnecessary health care costs. Several clinical and laboratory-based algorithms have been proposed for the same. Hospital Antibiotic Stewardship Programs and Infection Control teams generally monitor antibiotic usage and de-escalation strategies.

FURTHER READING

1. Balas MC, Burke WJ, Gannon D, et al. Implementing the awakening and breathing coordination, delirium monitoring/management, and early exercise/mobility bundle into everyday care: opportunities, challenges, and lessons learned for implementing the ICU Pain, Agitation, and Delirium Guidelines. Crit Care Med. 2013; 41:S116-S127.
2. Barlam TF, Cosgrove SE, Abbo LM, et al. Implementing an Antibiotic Stewardship Program: Guidelines by the Infectious Diseases Society of America and the Society for Healthcare Epidemiology of America. Clin Infect Dis. 2016;62:e51.
3. Barr J, Fraser GL, Puntillo K, et al. Clinical practice guidelines for the management of pain, agitation, and delirium in adult patients in the intensive care unit. Crit Care Med. 2013;41:263.
4. Ely EW, Inouye SK, Bernanrd GR, et al. Delirium in mechanically ventilated patients: validity and reliability of the confusion assessment method for the intensive care unit (CAM-ICU). J Am Med Assoc. 2001;286:2703-10.
5. Gordon H. Guyatt, Elie A. Akl, et al. Antithrombotic Therapy and Prevention of Thrombosis, 9th ed: American College of Chest Physicians Evidence-based Clinical Practice Guidelines. Chest. 2012;141(2_suppl):7S-47S.
6. McClave S, Taylor B, Martindale R, Warren M, Johnson D, Braun-Schweig C, et al. Guidelines for the Provision and Assessment of Nutrition Support Therapy in the Adult Critically Ill Patient: Society of Critical Care Medicine (SCCM) and American Society for Parenteral and Enteral Nutrition (ASPEN). Journal of Parenteral and Enteral Nutrition. 2016;40(2):159-211.
7. NICE-SUGAR Study Investigators, F*in*fer S, Chittock DR, et al. Intensive versus conventional glucose control in critically ill patients. N Engl J Med. 2009;360:1283.
8. Norma AM, Rita AF, et al. Head-of-Bed Elevation in Critically Ill Patients: A Review Crit Care Nurse. 2013;33:53-67.
9. Spirt MJ, Stanley S. Update on stress ulcer prophylaxis in critically ill patients. Crit Care Nurse. 2006;26:18.
10. Vincent JL. Give your patient a fast hug (at least) once a day. Crit Care Med. 2005;33(6):1225-9. Review.
11. Vincent WR 3rd, Hatton KW. Critically ill patients need "FAST HUGS BID" (an updated mnemonic). Crit Care Med. 2009; 37(7): 2326-7.

8

CHAPTER

Delirium in the Intensive Care Unit

Praveen Venishetty, Raymond D Savio

Critically-ill patients are at risk of developing various changes in neurological status which may be a manifestation of their basic disease state or of a new neurological injury. Early identification and appropriate management of these states can help in reducing the morbidity and mortality and the intensive care unit (ICU).

EPIDEMIOLOGY AND PROGNOSTIC SIGNIFICANCE

Delirium is one of the more common neurological states that is encountered in the ICU. It is defined by the American psychiatric Association as "a disturbance of consciousness that develops over a short period of time, fluctuates and is associated with perceptual changes such as hallucinations". One multicenter study for delirium had shown an incidence rate of 32.3%. The prevalence is lower in non-intubated patients (20%) compared to the intubated (83%). Akhilesh and colleagues had shown an incidence and prevalence rate of 24.4% and 53.6% respectively in an Indian ICU. It is also associated with adverse prognosis as it is shown to increase the ICU mortality by 2.5 fold and six month mortality by 3.2 fold (Fig. 1).

Thus, prevention, early recognition and appropriate management is of paramount importance.

Delirium is classified into three types (Table 1), hyperactive, hypoactive and mixed. Of all the three, hypoactive is the most common and the most unrecognized variety. It is often misdiagnosed as depressive illness. Hyperactive delirium is easily recognizable since the patients are agitated and restless but is least common of the three. In the mixed form patients alternate between both ends of the spectrum.

Anticipation of delirium can be done by risk identification, which therefore will help in early recognition and prompt management of this disorder. An easier way to remember the risk factors is with the mnemonic I *Watch Death* and *Delirium* (Table 2).

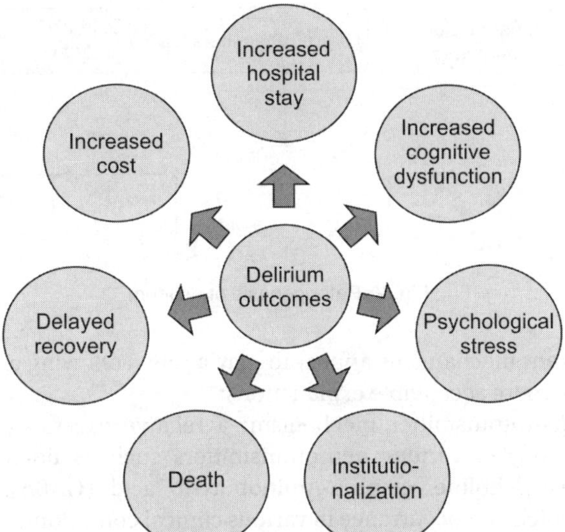

Fig. 1: Delirium outcomes

Table 1: Types of delirium

Type	*Clinical features*	*Incidence*
Hyperactive	Aggressive, restless, combative noncooperative	<5%, example alcohol withdrawl
Hypoactive	Calm, cooperative, lethargic, somnolent	45–64%, most common in ICU
Mixed	Features of both the above alternating	6–55% in ICU

Table 2: Precipitating factors for delirium in ICU

I Watch Death	*Delirium*
Infection	Drugs
Withdrawal	Electrolyte and physiologic abnormalities
Acute metabolic	Lack of drugs (withdrawal)
Trauma/pain	Infection
CNS pathology	Reduced sensory input (deafness, blindness)
Deficiency states (Vitamin B_{12}, Thiamine)	Intracranial problems
Endocrinopathy (Thyroid, adrenal)	Urinary retention
Acute vascular (Hypertension, shock)	Myocardial problems
Toxin/drugs	
Heavy metals	

PATHOPHYSIOLOGY (FIG. 2)

Multiple hypothesis have been put forward in various studies to explain the pathophysiological basis of delirium. However none of them appear to be applicable in all situations and

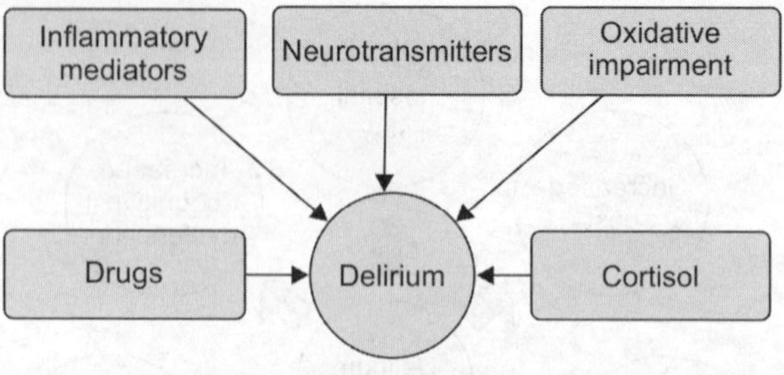

Fig. 2: Pathogenesis of delirium

different mechanisms appear to play a role. Following are few of the more acceptable explanations:

1. Neurotransmitter mechanism: a relative excess or deficiency of various neurotransmitters such as dopamine, acetylcholine, gamma-Aminobutyric acid (GABA), etc., which is a occurrence in various clinical conditions.
2. Inflammatory mediators: various acute phase reactants and mediators which initiate and perpetuate the inflammatory process that damage the endothelial covering and microvascular damage in central nervous system. For example, TNF-α, IL-1, cytokines and chemokines.
3. Oxidative metabolism: impaired oxidative metabolism secondary to inflammatory process and microvascular damage leading to cerebrovascular insufficiency.
4. Cortisol excess: excess cortisol during the stressful states as does occur in various diseases and infections itself has deleterious effects on neurons.
5. Neutral amino acid: availability of neutral amino acids is increased in stressful states. When they reach above their critical levels they cross blood brain barrier and have an effect on neuronal function. Tryptophan and phenylalanine are among the most studied. An increase in their levels in brain leads to increased levels of dopamine and norepinephrine which are implicated in pathogenesis of delirium.
6. Drugs: Benzodiazepines, Opioids, Dopaminergics, serotonergics, anticholinergics, H_2 blockers, steroids, metoclopramide, etc. have all been implicated in the causation of delirium.

WHEN TO SUSPECT?

Any patient with the above said risk factors and acute change in mental state should be suspected of having delirium based on arousability. The gold standard for delirium assessment is Delirium Observation Screening Scale (DOSS) mentioned in DSM-IV criteria which is 25 point scale and is very cumbersome. Recently three validated scales with good agreement with the DOSS scale and which can be easily performed bedside within 1–2 minutes have been developed. These are CAM-ICU, ICDSC and NEECHAM scale. The CAM-ICU scale is by far the most commonly used (Figs 3 and 4).

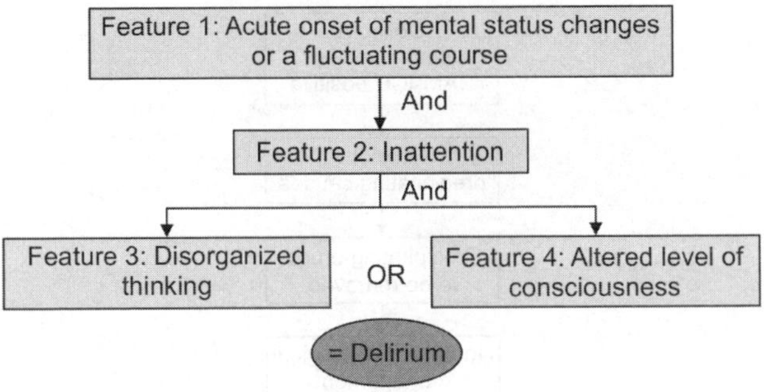

Fig. 3: Diagnosis of delirium

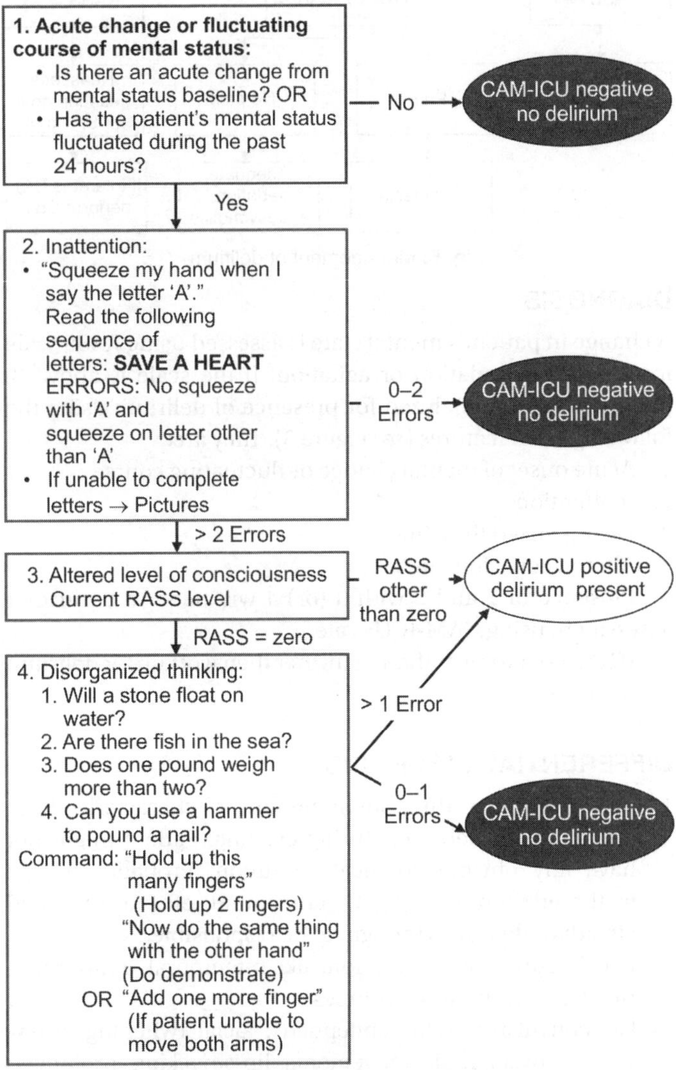

Fig. 4: CAM–ICU assessment for delirium
Abbreviation: RASS, Richmond Agitation-Sedation Scale.

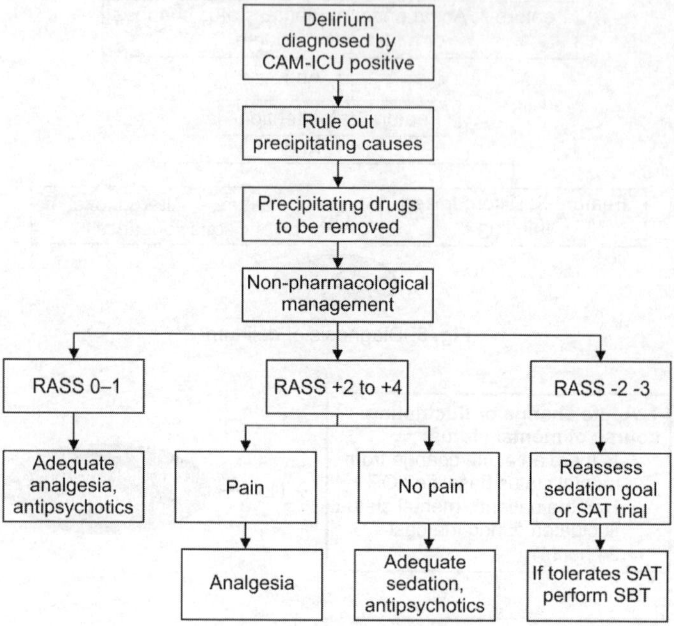

Fig. 5: Management of delirium

DIAGNOSIS

A change in patient's mental state is assessed using RASS scale for amount of sedation or agitation. If the scale is above–3, patient is further analyzed for presence of delirium using the following set of features (*see* Figure 3). They are:

1. Acute onset of mental change or fluctuating course
2. Inattention
3. Disorganized thinking
4. Altered consciousness.

Presence of 1 and 2 with 3 (or) 4 will need to be further assessment using CAM-ICU scale.

If RASS scale is less than –4 further then workup for delirium is not needed.

DIFFERENTIAL DIAGNOSIS

1. Sun downing: This phenomenon is characterized by alterations in behavior during evening. Patient might not have any obvious medical condition. Probably change in the environment (light, staff, sound, etc.) or impaired circadian rhythm is thought to be responsible.
2. Focal neurological conditions like bitemporal, temporoparietal and occipital syndromes.
3. Nonconvulsive status epilepticus: facial twitching, unexplained nystagmoid movements, lip smacking, prolonged postictal state, acute aphasia, unexplained confusional state.
4. Dementia: features of fluctuating mental state are present but insidious and prolonged in nature.

Table 3: Preventing delirium in ICU

Intervention	*Improved delirium outcomes*	*Other improved outcomes*
Awakening and breathing coordination	Shorter coma duration	Shorter MV Shorter length of stay Improved 1 year survival
Choice of sedative agents	Lower prevalence of delirium Shorter duration of brain dysfunction	Shorter MV Greater sedation accuracy
Delirium monitoring and management	Increased detection of delirium	
Early mobility and exercise	Shorter delirium duration	Increased return to independence Shorter ICU stay Decreased re-hospitalization

Source: Critical Care Clinics 2014.

Prevention of Delirium

Recently Brummel and colleagues devised a combined approach mechanism for the prevention of delirium, especially in ICU patients. The 'ABCDE' is a comprehensive approach for prevention and early management of delirium in ICU patients and includes in Figure 5 and Table 3.

- **A**wakening and **B**reathing coordination
- **C**hoice of sedative agents
- **D**elirium monitoring and management
- **E**arly mobility and exercise.

Awakening and Breathing Coordination

The importance of daily awakening (sedation interruption) coupled with SBT for patients receiving mechanical ventilation has been proved beyond doubt. This clearly decreases number of days on MV, ICU length of stay and mortality.

Choice of Sedative Agents

1. Stop benzodiazepines if present at the earliest
2. Titrate to the minimum level of sedation (mandatory to document level of sedation at all times)
3. Change the sedative drugs if needed.

Delirium Monitoring and Management

1. Early identification of change in mental status
2. Performing CAM-ICU or other scales to confirm the presence of delirium
3. Treating the precipitating factor after considering and ruling out other differential diagnosis.

Early Mobility and Exercise

1. Daily passive range of movements
2. Physiotherapy
3. Early ambulation.

Investigation to Rule Out Alternative Diagnosis

1. Complete blood picture and cultures of appropriate samples to rule out infections
2. ABG levels for hypoxia, metabolic acidosis, hypercapnia
3. Liver function tests
4. Kidney function tests to rule out uremia and renal failure
5. Drug levels for precipitating drugs
6. Brain imaging if needed to rule out any organic insult
7. Lumbar puncture when CNS infection is suspected
8. Electroencephalogram (EEG) for ictal, postictal, or nonconvulsive status epilepticus.

Management

Management of delirium begins with prompt identification and mitigation of precipitating factors. All differential diagnosis are to be considered and suitable nonpharmacological measures implemented before embarking on pharmacological measures.

Nonpharmacological Management Includes

1. Improved communication
2. Frequent meet with relatives
3. Music or television with a sense of information going around the world
4. Adequacy of nursing staff and frequent verbal communication
5. Proper sleep hygiene with light switching on and off during the day and night respectively to provide them a sense of diurnal variation
6. Control excessive noises in ICU as much as possible.

Pharmacological Management

- Control adequate tissue perfusion by correcting volume deficit and maintaining normal BP
- Titrate oxygen supplementation for maintaining SpO_2 >88%
- Electrolyte and metabolic corrections as needed
- Stop precipitating drugs if present which include opioids, benzodiazepines, serotonergics, steroids, etc.
- Antipsychotics.

None of the drugs are FDA approved for ICU delirium and the current recommendations are only consensus statements from various studies.

Haloperidol

It is a typical antipsychotic given at dosage of 2–5 mg initially followed by 2.5 mg every 6th hourly according to the need. Dose should not exceed beyond 20 mg/day. QT prolongation should be watched for carefully.

Dexmedetomidine

It is newer α_2 agonist which has been compared with benzodiazepines, especially lorazepam. Two studies namely MENDS trial and SEDCOM trial have proven its efficacy over benzodiazepines in preventing and treating delirium. It is given at a dose of 1 μg/kg bolus over 10–20 minutes followed by 0.2–0.7 μg/kg infusion. Bradycardia and hypotension are the important side effects to be careful about.

FURTHER READING

1. American Psychiatric Association. Diagnostic and Statistical Manual of Mental Disorders DSMIVTR, 4th edn (Text Revision).Washington DC: American Psychiatric Association; 2000.
2. Burgeron, et al. Intensive care delirium screening check list: evaluation of a new screening tool, Intensive Care Med. 2001;27:859-64.
3. Cavallazzi R, Saad M, Marik PE, et al. Delirium in the ICU: an overview. Ann Intensive Care. 2012;2:49.
4. Ely EW, Inouye SK, Bernard GR, Gordon S, Francis J, May L, et al. Delirium in mechanically ventilated patients: validity and reliability of the confusion assessment method for the intensive care unit (CAM-ICU) JAMA. 2001;286(21):2703-10.
5. Girard TD, Kress JP, Fuchs BD, et al. Efficacy and safety of a paired sedation and ventilator weaning protocol for mechanically ventilated patients in intensive care (Awakening and Breathing Controlled trial): a randomised controlled trial. Lancet. 2008;371:126-34.
6. Girard TD, Pandharipande PP, Ely EW. Delirium in the intensive care unit. Crit Care. 2008;12(Suppl 3):S3.
7. Morandi A, Brummel NE, Ely EW. Sedation, delirium and mechanical ventilation: the 'ABCDE' approach. Curr Opin Crit Care. 2011; 17(1):43-9.
8. Salluh JI, Soares M, Teles JM, et al. Epidemiology in Critical Care Study Group. Delirium epidemiology in critical care (DECCA): an international study. Crit Care. 2010;14(6):R210.
9. Sessler CN, Gosnell MS, Grap MJ, Brophy GM, O'neal PV, Keane KA, et al. "The Richmond Agitation–Sedation Scale", American Journal of Respiratory and Critical Care Medicine. 2002; 166(10):1338-44.
10 Sharma A, Malhotra S, Grover S, Jindal SK, et al. Incidence, prevalence, risk factor and outcome of delirium in intensive care unit: a study from India. Gen Hos Psy. 2012;39(6):639-46.
11. Van RB, Schuurmans MJ, Shortridge-Baggett LM, Truijen S, Elseviers M, Bossaert L. A comparison of the CAM-ICU and the NEECHAM Confusion Scale in intensive care delirium assessment: an observational study in non-intubated patients. Crit Care. 2008;12(1):R16.

9

CHAPTER

Sedation in the Critically Ill

Raymond D Savio

Maintaining an optimal level of comfort and safety for critically ill patients is a universal goal for critical care practitioners.

ANALGESIA

Intensive care unit (ICU) patients commonly have pain and physical discomfort from obvious factors, such as pre-existing diseases, invasive procedures, or trauma. Pain and discomfort can also be caused by monitoring and therapeutic devices (such as catheters, drains, ET tubes), routine nursing care (suction, physiotherapy, dressing changes, and patient mobilization), and prolonged immobility. Effective analgesia may diminish pulmonary complications in postoperative patients.

ANALGESIA THERAPY

Non-pharmacologic interventions including attention to proper positioning, stabilization of fractures, and elimination of irritating physical stimulation (e.g. proper positioning of ventilator tubing to avoid traction on the endotracheal tube) are important to maintain patient comfort. Application of heat or cold therapy may be useful.

Pharmacologic therapies include opioids, nonsteroidal anti-inflammatory drugs (NSAIDs), and acetaminophen. The analgesic agents most commonly used in ICU patients (fentanyl, morphine) are addressed later.

OPIOID ADMINISTRATION TECHNIQUES

Preventing pain is more effective than treating established pain. Analgesics should be administered on a continuous or scheduled intermittent basis, with supplemental bolus doses as required (Table 1). Intravenous administration usually requires lower doses than intramuscular administration. Intramuscular administration is not recommended in hemodynamically unstable patients because of altered perfusion and variable absorption. When a continuous infusion was used, a protocol incorporating daily awakening from analgesia and sedation allowed more effective analgesic titration and a lower total dose

Table 1: Pharmacology of selected analgesics

Agent	*Equianalgesic dose (IV)*	*Half-life*	*Metabolic pathway*	*Active metabolites*	*Adverse effects*
Fentanyl	200 μg	1.5–6 h	Oxidation	No metabolite	Rigidity
Morphine	10 mg	3–7 h	Glucuronidation	Yes	Histamine release
Remifentanil	Bolus not recommended	3–10 min	Plasma esterase	None	Risk of GI bleeding

of morphine. Daily awakening was associated with a shorter duration of ventilation and ICU stay. A pain management plan and therapy goal should be established for each patient and reevaluated as the clinical condition changes.

SEDATION ASSESSMENT

Frequent assessment of the degree of sedation or agitation may facilitate the titration of sedatives to predetermined endpoints. An ideal sedation scale should provide data that are simple to compute and record accurately, describe the degree of sedation or agitation within well-defined categories and guide the titration of therapy.

Many scales are available, but a true gold standard scale has not been established. None of the scales have been tested for their ability to detect a patient's response to changes in sedative therapy, dosage, or withdrawal. However, a defined sedation goal, using the Ramsay scale and a protocol-driven sedation plan, was shown to reduce the duration of mechanical ventilation and length of stay. The Riker Sedation-Agitation Scale (SAS) was the first scale proven to be reliable and valid in critically ill adults.

The Ramsay scale measures three levels of awake states and three levels of sleep states (Table 2). It has been shown to have an acceptable inter observer reliability. The appropriate target level of sedation will primarily depend on a patient's acute disease process and any therapeutic and supportive interventions required. A common target level of sedation in the ICU is a calm patient that can be easily aroused with maintenance of the normal sleep-wake cycle, but some may require deep levels of sedation to facilitate mechanical ventilation.

Table 2: Ramsay sedation scale

Score	*Response*
1	Anxious or restless or both
2	Cooperative, orientated and tranquil
3	Responding to commands
4	Brisk response to stimulus
5	Sluggish response to stimulus
6	No response to stimulus please convert to tabular format

SEDATION THERAPY

Benzodiazepines

Benzodiazepines are sedatives and hypnotics that block potentially unpleasant experiences (anterograde amnesia) but do not induce retrograde amnesia. Elderly patients exhibit slower clearance of benzodiazepines or their active metabolites and have a larger volume of drug distribution, contributing to a marked prolongation of elimination.

Midazolam has a rapid onset and short duration with single doses, similar to diazepam. The rapid onset of midazolam makes it preferable for treating acutely agitated patients. Accumulation and prolonged sedative effects have been reported in critically ill patients using midazolam who are obese or have a low albumin level or renal failure. Prolonged sedation may be caused by the accumulation of an active metabolite, alpha-hydroxymidazolam in patients with renal insufficiency. The routine use of a benzodiazepine antagonist, such as flumazenil, is not recommended

Propofol

Propofol is an intravenous, general anesthetic agent. However, sedative and hypnotic properties can be demonstrated at lower doses. Compared with benzodiazepines, propofol produces a similar degree of amnesia at equisedative doses in volunteers. In a clinical trial of ICU patients, propofol did not produce amnesia as often as midazolam. Like the benzodiazepines, propofol has no analgesic properties.

Propofol has a rapid onset and short duration of sedation once discontinued. While most of the early literature documents the comparatively rapid resolution of sedation after propofol infusions, a slightly longer recovery has been reported after more than 12 hours of infusion. No changes in kinetic parameters have been reported in patients with renal or hepatic dysfunction. Propofol is available as an emulsion in a phospholipid vehicle, which provides 1.1 kcal/mL from fat and should be counted as a caloric source. Long-term or high-dose infusions may result in hypertriglyceridemia. Other adverse effects most commonly seen with propofol include hypotension, bradycardia, and pain upon peripheral venous injection.

The hypotension is dose related and more frequent after bolus dose administration.

Propofol requires a dedicated line for continuous infusion because of the potential for drug incompatibility and infection. While propofol appears to possess anticonvulsant activity, excitatory phenomena, such as myoclonus, have been observed. Propofol has been used to sedate neurosurgical patients to reduce elevated intracranial pressure (ICP). The rapid awakening from propofol allows interruption of the infusion for neurologic assessment.

Central Alpha-agonists

Clonidine has been used to augment the effects of general anesthetics and narcotics and to treat drug withdrawal syndromes in the ICU. The more selective α-2 agonist, dexmedetomidine, was recently approved for use as a sedative with analgesic-sparing activity for short-term use (<24 hours) in patients who are receiving mechanical ventilation. Patients remain sedated when undisturbed, but arouse readily with gentle stimulation. Dexmedetomidine reduces concurrent analgesic and sedative requirements and produces anxiolytic effects comparable to benzodiazepines. Rapid administration of dexmedetomidine may produce transient elevations in blood pressure. Patients maintained on dexmedetomidine may develop bradycardia and hypotension, especially in the presence of intravascular volume depletion or high sympathetic tone. The role of this new agent in the sedation of ICU patients remains to be determined.

3

Section

Patient Monitoring

SECTION EDITOR: Supradip Ghosh

10

CHAPTER

Hemodynamics in Critical Care

Supradip Ghosh

INTRODUCTION

Adequate flow of blood, delivery of oxygen and nutrients to tissue is essential for survival. The term hemodynamics is derived from two Greek words—"Heme" or blood and "dynamus" or movement, meaning the movement of blood within the circulatory system. Hemodynamic instability is common in critically-ill patients. Failure to recognize early signs of hemodynamic instability leads to multiple organ dysfunction syndrome (MODS) and eventually adverse outcome. Hemodynamic monitoring is necessary for the early recognition of global and regional tissue perfusion, timely and adequate correction of instability and halt the progression to MODS. A bedside nurse should be able to monitor and interpret basic hemodynamic data obtained from a patient.

Learning Objectives

1. Terminologies used in hemodynamic monitoring.
2. Steps of hemodynamic monitoring.
3. Setting up invasive monitoring devices—central venous pressure, arterial pressure and pulmonary artery catheter.
4. Interpretation of data obtained.

Some Terminologies You must know

Stroke Volume (SV)

Stroke volume is the volume of blood ejected in one ventricular systole. Normal value is 60–120 mL. In normal physiology, ventricles can only eject the amount of blood returned to them from systemic or pulmonary veins, also known as venous return. For example, LVSV or RVSV [LV = Left ventricle. RV = Right ventricle]. SV depends on three variables—Preload, contractility of cardiac myocyte and afterload.

Preload

Preload is the length of ventricular muscle fiber prior to contraction and dependent on ventricular filling or venous return. It is indirectly reflected by ventricular filling pressure, e.g. central venous pressure (CVP) for right ventricle and pulmonary artery occlusion pressure (PAOP) for left ventricle.

Contractility

Intrinsic ability of the cardiac muscle to develop force for a given muscle length. Ejection fraction measured by echocardiography may be used as a surrogate of contractility.

Afterload

Afterload is the tension against which ventricle must contract. Arterial pressure or vascular resistance reflects the afterload of a given ventricle.

Stroke Volume Index (SVI)

SV corrected for body size. Normal value for SVI is 2.5–3.5 mL/m^2 BSA. [BSA – Body Surface Area].

End-diastolic Volume (EDV)

Total volume of blood accumulated in a ventricle at the end of ventricular diastole.

End-systolic Volume (ESV)

Volume of blood that remains in a ventricle at the end of systole.

$$SV = EDV - ESV$$

Ejection Fraction (EF)

Percentage of blood that is pumped out of the ventricle during systole. Its normal value is 50–75%. Ejection fraction can be easily measured at the bedside by an echocardiographic examination. For example, LVEF or RVEF.

$$EF (\%) = (EDV - ESV)/EDV \times 100$$

Cardiac Output (CO)

Cardiac output is defined as amount of blood ejected from a ventricle per minute. Normal value for CO is 4–8 L/min.

$$CO = SV \times HR \text{ [HR = Heart Rate]}$$

Cardiac Index (CI)

Cardiac output corrected for difference in body size. Normal value for CI is 2.5–4 L/min/m^2.

Systemic Vascular Resistance (SVR)

SVR is defined as the resistance in the systemic vasculature against the blood flow from left ventricle. It depends upon systemic vascular tone. Normal value for SVR is 800–1400 dynes/sec/cm^{-5}.

Pulmonary Vascular Resistance (PVR)

PVR is defined as the resistance in the pulmonary vasculature against the blood flow from right ventricle or pulmonary vascular tone. Normal value for PVR is 120–250 dynes/sec/cm^{-5}.

Understanding Blood Pressure

Blood pressure is the lateral pressure created by the column of blood over the vessel wall. It is the product of cardiac output and systemic vascular resistance. It may be measured non-invasively with a cuff placed around a limb and attached to a sphygmomanometer or an oscillometric device, or it can be measured invasively using an indwelling catheter in an artery. Systolic blood pressure (SBP) is the peak pressure recorded during systole. Diastolic blood pressure (DBP) is the minimal pressure measured during diastole. Mean arterial pressure (MAP) is the average pressure exerted throughout the cardiac cycle.

MAP = (2 X DBP + SBP)/3 [MAP is an approximation of organ perfusion pressure]

Pulse pressure (PP) = SBP – DBP [PP is a surrogate marker for stroke volume]

Steps of Hemodynamic Monitoring

Step 1: Clinical Assessment

Look for level of consciousness, skin temperature, skin color or any mottling, capillary refill, urine output, heart rate and blood pressure (non-invasive). A conscious patient with a warm handshake and having adequate urine output probably do not require any advance hemodynamic monitoring.

Step 2: Basic Monitoring and Assessment of Global Perfusion

A sick patient needs continuous monitoring of electrocardiogram for any arrhythmia, pulse oxymetry for oxygenation and perhaps invasive monitoring of blood pressure. Serum lactate can be monitored periodically to look for global tissue hypoperfusion. Mixed venous or central venous oxygen saturation monitoring may be useful parameter in selected patients.

Step 3: Assessment of Preload

In a hypotensive patient preload may be assessed to optimize the cardiac performance. There are certain static (e.g. CVP, PAOP, LVEDV) or dynamic parameters (e.g. pulse pressure variation, systolic pressure variation or inferior vena cava distensibility or superior vena cava collapsibility) to assess preload. A passive leg-raising maneuver may be performed for preload assessment.

Step 4: Cardiac Output Monitoring

Cardiac output is measured at the bedside by using various techniques like pulmonary Thermodilution (Pulmonary Artery Catheter), transpulmonary Thermodilution (PiCCO or VolumeView), indicator dilution (LiDCO), arterial pulse contour analysis (Vigileo or PiCCO or VolumeView) or echocardiography.

Step 5: Assessment of Contractility

Simplest way to assess the intrinsic contractility of the ventricle is to look for ejection fraction by echocardiography.

Invasive Hemodynamic Monitoring System

In general, invasive hemodynamic monitoring system requires following things as depicted in Figure 1.

Flush Solution

About 500 mL normal saline preferably in a self-collapsible bag (may have 500 units of heparin in each 500 mL NS). This will allow a small continuous flush of 1–3 mL/hour for patency and flushing when needed.

Pressure Bag

The bag should always be inflated to 300 mm Hg.

Pressure Tubing

This tubing is non-compliant tubing. Prior to insertion, the tubing should be flushed completely and all air bubbles eliminated. This fluid-filled tubing transmits the signal from the patient to the transducer, which then is translated to waveforms and values on the monitor.

Pressure Transducer

This is where the stopcock will be placed. This is where the mechanical wave signals are converted to electrical signal.

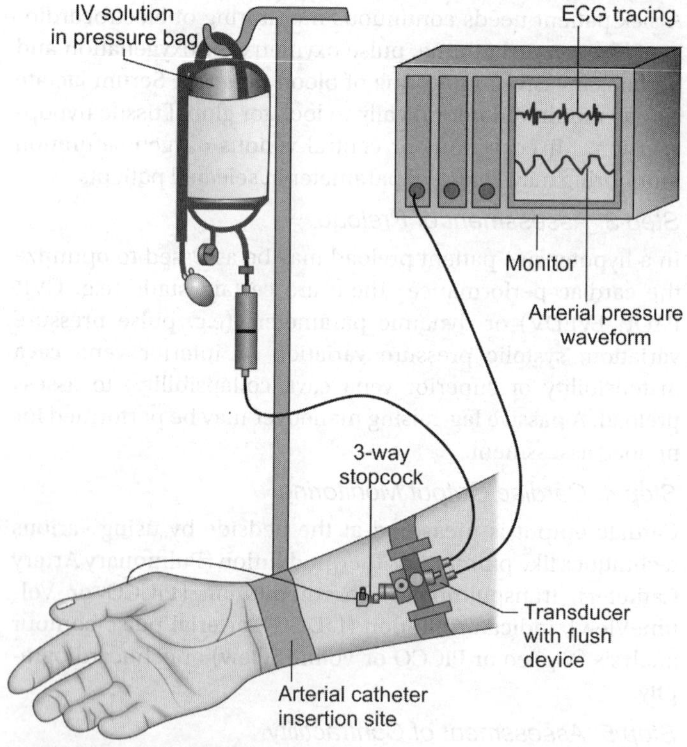

Fig. 1: Arterial line set up, the mechanical signal obtained from the arterial line is coverted to an electric signal by the transducer, filtered, amplified and displayed on the monitor

Stopcocks

Stopcocks are part of the pressure tubing. Place non-vented caps on the stopcocks as this will prevent air from entering the system.

Cables

Cables are plugged into the transducer as well as the module connected to the monitor.

Monitor

Display values and waveforms.

ENSURING ACCURACY

The transducer should be leveled with the phlebostatic axis, at the same level as the right atrium. It may be estimated by intersecting lines from the fourth intercostal space and the mid axillary line as shown in Figure 2.

Leveling should be done before and after connecting the pressure system to the patient, with every change in bed height or changes in the elevation of the head of the bed, with any significant change in patient's hemodynamic variables, and prior to zeroing and calibration. The reference port on the transducer should be open and the appropriate "zero" buttons on the bedside monitor should be pushed. Zeroing is performed to eliminate the effects of atmospheric pressure on the transducer. Zeroing should be performed before and after connecting the pressure system to the patient, with any leveling, and whenever there is a significant change in the hemodynamic variables. All values should be rated at the end of expiration to negate the effect of intrathoracic pressure.

Who Requires an Arterial Catheter?

1. Unstable blood pressure or anticipation of unstable blood pressure, e.g. patient in shock or prolonged surgery with anticipated changes in hemodynamics.
2. Use of rapidly acting vasoactive drugs; vasodilators, vasopressors, inotropes
3. Frequent sampling of arterial blood.
4. Presence of an intra-aortic balloon pump.
5. Patients with unreliable, or difficult to obtain, non-invasive BP, e.g. very obese patients.

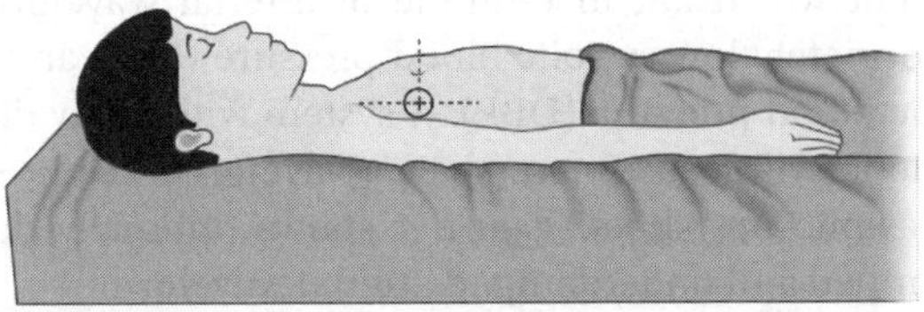

Fig. 2: Reference zero on the phlebostatic axis

Contraindications to Invasive Arterial Pressure Monitoring

There is no absolute contraindication to invasive arterial pressure monitoring. Some relative contraindications are:

1. Anticipation of thrombolytic therapy.
2. Severe peripheral vascular disease preventing catheter insertion.
3. Vascular anomalies—AV fistula, local aneurysm, local hematoma, Raynaud's disease.
4. Lack of collateral blood flow distally (e.g. radial artery previously used for coronary artery bypass surgery).

Sites for Arterial Cannulation

Radial, femoral and dorsalis pedis arteries are usual choice for arterial cannulation. Brachial artery is avoided, as it is an end-artery. Radial artery preferred, as it is superficial, easily compressible and has good collateral circulation.

Modified Allen's Test

This test was historically performed to test the patency of ipsilateral ulnar artery and collateral circulation of hand, before radial artery cannulation.

Step 1: Patient is asked to clench his/her fist.

Step 2: With both thumbs, the ulnar and radial arteries are simultaneously occluded.

Step 3: With pressure on, patient is asked to relax hand. Blanching of palm and fingers should occur.

Step 4: Now pressure is released on ulnar artery. There should be flushing within 5–15 seconds denoting patency of ulnar artery.

Interpretation

Positive modified Allen's test means it is safe to do radial cannulation.

COMPONENTS OF ARTERIAL WAVEFORMS (FIG. 3)

Abnormal Arterial Pressure Waveforms

Damping coefficient refers to how quickly the oscillating, fluid-filled system comes to rest. A system with a high damping coefficient will result in blunting of arterial waveform with inappropriately low systolic blood pressure (SBP) and higher diastolic blood pressure (DBP). A system with a low damping coefficient will cause too sharp waveforms with systolic and diastolic overshoot. Figure 4 shows optimally damped, overdamped and underdamped arterial waveform.

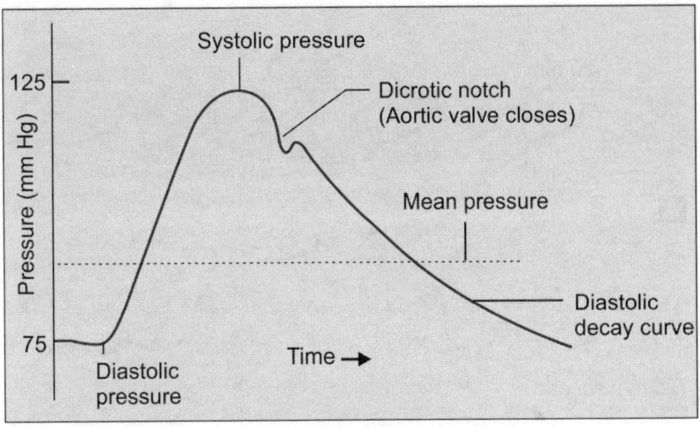

Fig. 3: Components of arterial waveforms, the area under the curve equals the cardiac output

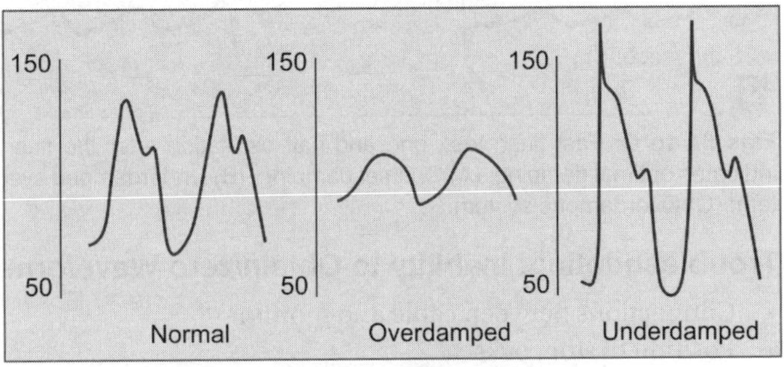

Fig. 4: Effect of damping

Checking the System—Fast Flush Test

Opening the valve of the continuous flush device, acutely increase the pressure to 30 mL/hour. This acute rise in pressure within the system produces a square wave on the monitor. Closure of the valve generates a sinusoidal pressure wave of a given frequency and progressively decreasing amplitude. It will return to the baseline within one or two oscillations normally (Fig. 5A). If there are multiple small spikes at the down stroke of the waveform, the system is underdamped (Fig. 5B). If the number of oscillations are <2 the system is overdamped (Fig. 5C).

Troubleshooting: Damped Waveforms

- Check for the pressure of the bag. It should be inflated to 300 mm Hg
- Reposition the patient and do the leveling
- Verify appropriate scale
- Look for air bubble and aspirate the line
- Flush the system
- Check or replace module or cable.

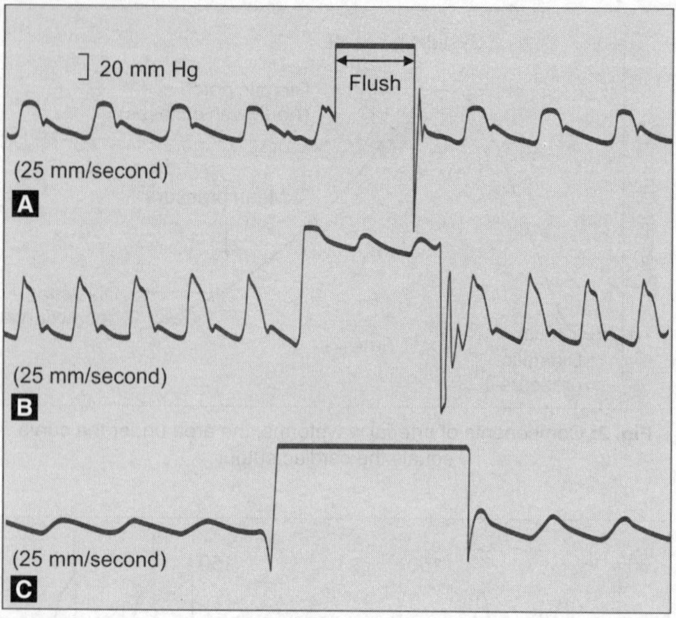

Figs 5A to C: Fast flush test, one and half oscillation after the flush indicates optimal damping. (A) Optimal damping; (B) Underdamped system; (C) Overdamped system

Troubleshooting: Inability to Obtain/zero Waveform

- Connections between cable and monitor
- Position of stopcocks
- Retry zeroing after above adjustments.

CENTRAL VENOUS PRESSURE

Who Requires a Central Venous Catheter?

1. Measurement of central venous pressure (providing catheter tip located proximal superior vena cava)
2. Infusion of vasoactive drugs, hyperosmolar fluids (including parenteral nutrition), irritant solutions, e.g. concentrated potassium solution or amiodarone.
3. Inability to obtain peripheral intravenous access
4. Hemodialysis, plasmapheresis, transvenous pacing.

Contraindications to Insertion of a Central Venous Catheter

1. Severe coagulopathy or anticipation of need for thrombolysis
2. Obvious infection of overlying skin
3. Thrombosis of superior vena cava or subclavian vein.

Central Venous Pressure (CVP) Waves

Why to Measure CVP?

1. CVP is presumed to be a surrogate marker for right ventricular preload. But this presumption has fallacies, as CVP is

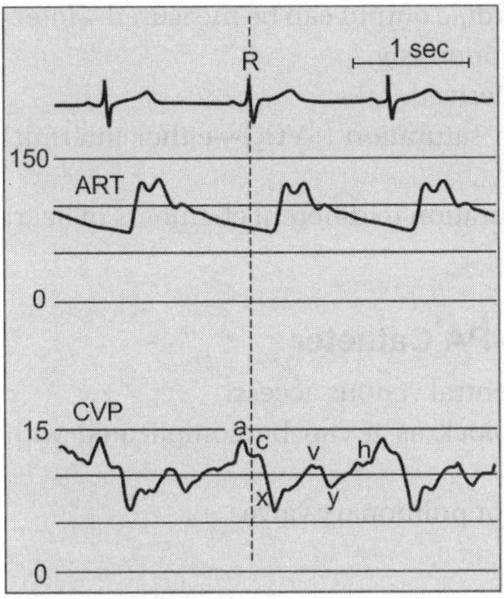

a-wave: RA contraction
c-wave: Tricuspid bulging during RV systole
x-decent: RA relaxation
v-wave: Atrial filling during RV systole
y-decent: Early RV filling
h-wave: Diastolic plateau
*Measurement of CVP is done at endexpiration

Fig. 6: Components of central venous pressure (CVP) waveform

influenced by many other factors, including Intrathoracic pressure changes (e.g. mechanical ventilation, pneumothorax), intra-abdominal pressure changes, compliance of right ventricle, pulmonary vascular resistance, etc. But CVP trending during fluid challenge may still be useful and may be utilized as a limit to further fluid challenge.

"Two-in-Five Rule": During fluid challenge continuously measure the CVP readings. If CVP rises to >5 cm H_2O during fluid challenge or >2 cm H_2O after the challenge, stop further fluid loading.

2. Classic CVP morphology can give clue to underlying disease process. For example, giant a-wave in tricuspid stenosis or giant v-wave in tricuspid regurgitation.

PULMONARY ARTERY CATHETER

Pulmonary artery catheter, still considered as the gold standard for hemodynamic monitoring, was developed by Dr HJ Swan and Dr W Ganz in 1970. With the availability of less invasive monitoring system and its futility in decreasing mortality in critically-ill patients has limited its use in modern ICU.
It is still being used in selected clinical conditions:

- Complicated cardiac and noncardiac surgery
- Situations where noninvasive techniques fail to give clue to hemodynamic compromise
- Diagnosis of intracardiac shunts
- Before heart-lung transplant.

What All Parameters You can Measure?

- Pressure: Right atrial pressure, right ventricular pressure, pulmonary artery pressure, pulmonary artery occlusion pressure (indirectly reflecting LA pressure) can be measured directly.

- Stroke volume and cardiac output can be measured—intermittently or semi-continuously.
- SVR and PVR can be derived.
- Mixed venous oxygen saturation (SVO_2)—either intermittently or continuously.
- Change in oxygen saturation in different chambers of heart to diagnose shunt.

Contraindications to PA Catheter

- Contraindication to central venous access.
- Left bundle branch block as it can be complicated with complete AV block.
- Mechanical tricuspid or pulmonary valves.

Risks Involved

- Complications of central venous access.
- Mechanical injury to cardiac structures.
- Pulmonary artery rupture and pulmonary infarction—more common if balloon remains inflated for more than 15 seconds.
- Arrhythmias including life-threatening ventricular tachycardias and complete AV block.
- Coiling of catheter in the RA (more common in tricuspid regurgitation) or right ventricle (dilated RV or low output state).

ROLE OF NURSES

1. To assist the physicians during insertion of invasive devices for hemodynamic monitoring. Nurse need to ensure that strict aseptic precautions are followed during insertion.
2. Setting up the monitoring system including leveling and zeroing.
3. Maintenance of devices—following infection control practices, ensuring patency of the device, periodic dressing changes.
4. Ensuring the accuracy of the data obtained.
5. Interpreting the data at the bedside and alarming the physician about any abnormal data.
6. Ensuring that invasive lines are not being kept for longer than required.

11

CHAPTER

Pulse Oximetry and End-tidal Carbon Dioxide Monitoring

Supradip Ghosh

PULSE OXIMETRY

Tissue needs oxygen for survival and oxygen is supplied to the tissue by the arterial blood, mostly by the hemoglobin contained inside the red blood cells (RBCs). Ensuring adequate supply of oxygen to the tissues, is the most important goal of modern day intensive care. Continuous monitoring of arterial blood saturation using pulse oximetry has thus become the standard of care in the ICU.

What is Oxygen Saturation?

One molecule of hemoglobin can carry up to four molecules of oxygen after which it is described as "saturated" with oxygen. Percentage of hemoglobin molecule saturated with oxygen in the blood is called oxygen saturation. SaO_2 is oxygen saturation measured by the blood gas machine and SpO_2 is oxygen saturation estimated from the pulse oximetry from the periphery (the letter p stands for peripheral). A healthy individual with normal lungs, breathing air at sea level, will have an arterial oxygen saturation of 95–100%. Extremes of altitude will affect these numbers. Venous blood that is collected from the tissues contains less oxygen and normally has a saturation of around 75%.

Principles of Pulse Oximetry

Pulse oximeter determines the SpO_2 by applying the principle of differential absorption of two specific light wavelengths: 660 nm (red) and 940 nm (infrared) by the arterial blood. The ratio of absorbencies at the wavelengths is calibrated empirically against direct measurements of SaO_2 and the resulting calibration curve is used to generate estimated of arterial saturation or SpO_2 as a percentage, along with the heart rate and a plethysmographic waveform. Interpreting this waveform is essential in distinguishing a true oximeter signal from an artifact.

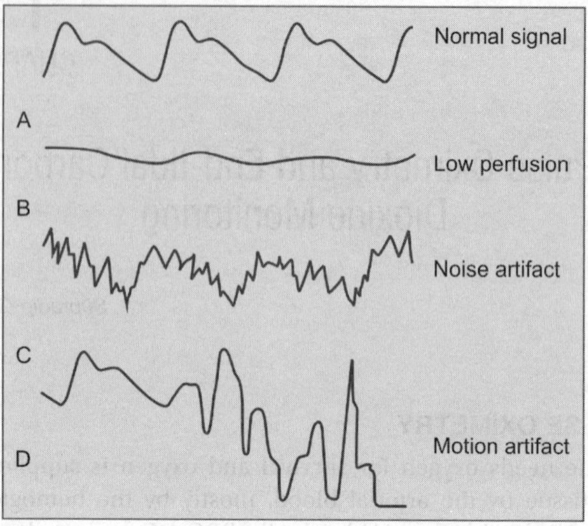

Fig. 1: Normal waveform and artifacts

Information Derived from a Pulse Oximeter

1. Continuous display of SpO_2.
2. Heart rate in beats per minute averaged over 5 to 20 seconds.
3. Plethysmographic signals or pulse waveform: May indicate the strength of the pulse and how well the tissues are perfused. The signal strength falls if the circulation becomes inadequate. (Fig. 1).

How to use the Pulse Oximeter?

- Select the appropriate probe with particular attention to correct sizing and the area of application finger, toe or ear. Make sure the area is clean prior to applying the probe. Remove any nail polish.
- Make sure the probe fits easily without being too loose or too tight.
- If possible, avoid the arm being used for blood pressure monitoring, as cuff inflation will interrupt the pulse oximeter signal.
- Look for the displayed pulse indicator that shows that the machine has detected a pulse. Without a pulse signal, any readings are meaningless.
- Like all machines, oximeters may occasionally give a false reading. Placing it on your own finger can check function of the oximeter probe.
- Always make sure the alarms are on.

Limitations of Pulse Oximetry

- **Physiological limitation:** Pulse oximetry reading correlates well with SaO_2 when oxygen saturation is between 70 and 100%. SpO_2 is physiologically related partial pressure of oxygen (PaO_2) in the blood according to oxyhemoglobin dissociation curve. But at both high level of PaO_2 and level below 60 mm Hg, the correlation between SpO_2 and PaO_2 becomes unpredictable because of the sigmoid nature of the curve.

- **Low perfusion state:** In state of low cardiac output, vasoconstriction or hypothermia sensor fails to distinguish true signal from background noise.
- **Dyshemoglobinemia:** Pulse oximetry readings are unreliable in the presence of significant level of methemoglobin and carboxyhemoglobin.
- Presence of certain dye in the blood like methylene blue (used in methemoglobinemia) or indocyanine green or indigo carmine.
- **Dark pigmentation and nail polish:** Gives falsely low reading.

Role of Nurses

- Ensure the technical quality of pulse oximetry signal.
- Taking care of the equipments, particularly the probe. Probe may be cleaned with alcohol swab.
- For best signals wrap the patient's hand that has the probe.
- Place the pulse oximeter on the finger of the opposite arm to where the blood pressure is taken.
- Correlate the heart rate displayed by SpO_2 reading to the heart rate from the ECG monitor. If they do not correlate, it may indicate not all heart beats are being sensed and the SpO_2 readings may be erroneous.
- When not in use the cable should not be tightly coiled to avoid damage to the cable.
- Maintain SpO_2 >92% in critically ill patients, unless specified otherwise.

END-TIDAL CARBON DIOXIDE MONITORING

End-tidal carbon dioxide monitoring ($ETCO_2$) refers to the noninvasive measurement of exhaled carbon dioxide, commonly used in intubated patients receiving mechanical ventilation. The term "capnometry" refers to the measurement and display of the concentration of exhaled carbon dioxide either as a percentage (%) or as partial pressure in millimeters of mercury (mm Hg). If the gas measuring device also includes a visual waveform recording the concentrations of inhaled and exhaled carbon dioxide, the instrument is called a capnograph.

Measurement of End-tidal Carbon Dioxide

Depending on the type of equipment used, the concentration of inspired and expired carbon dioxide can be measured directly at the patient-ventilator interface (mainstream sensor),

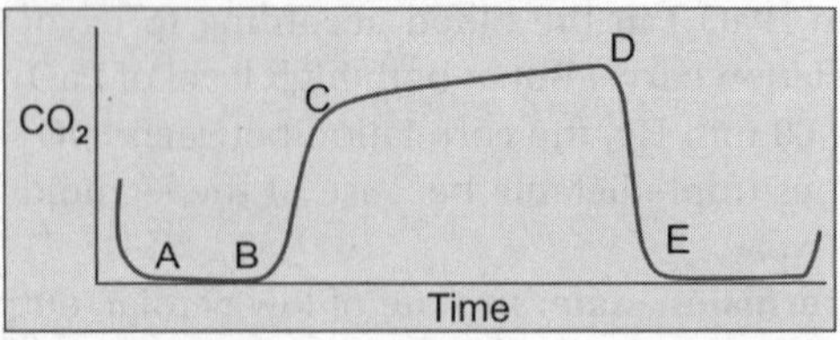

Fig. 2: Capnogram—the expired CO_2 levels in a breath cycle

or a sample of gases can be transported by a narrow bore tube to the bedside monitor (sidestream). Concentrations of expired carbon dioxide from the patient's airway are typically determined by using infrared light. With this method, the absorption of carbon dioxide molecules exposed to various wavelengths of light within a sample chamber or cell is measured. A photodetector then compares the relative amount of light absorbed by the sample with the amount absorbed by a gas that is free of carbon dioxide. The difference between the two represents the concentration of carbon dioxide.

The airway adapter or sampling port should be as close as possible to the patient's airway. It is kept upright to prevent water and secretions to pool at the bottom of the adapter.

Always support the positioning of the airway adapter or sampling port to minimize pull or weight on the patient's airway.

Typical normal carbon dioxide waveform. A to B, exhalation of carbon dioxide-free gas from dead space. B to C, combination of dead space and alveolar gases. C to D, exhalation of mostly alveolar gas (alveolar plateau). D, end-tidal point, that is, exhalation of carbon dioxide at maximum point. D to E, inspiration begins and carbon dioxide concentration rapidly falls to baseline or zero.

Continuous capnography detects small changes in patient's lung conditins such as extent of venous admixture or shunting or recruitment of alveoli after application of positive end-respiratory pressure (PEEP). Usually $EtCO_2$ is 1–5 mm Hg less than $PaCO_2$. However levels are affected by conditions common in the ICU such as hypovolemia, elevated alveolar pressure produced by high PEEP, sepsis, alterations in temperature and pulmonary embolism to name a few. So interpretation of $EtCO_2$ levels must factor in these limitations.

Despite these limitations $EtCO_2$ has many uses:

- It is the best method to confirm correct placement of endotracheal tube and for early detection of leaks and disconnections in the ventilator circuit.
- It is helpful in monitoring ventilation when the patient is in deep sedation and also during weaning.
- It is very useful to assess the effectiveness of cardiac compressions during cardiopulmonary resuscitation (CPR).

4

Section

Mechanical Ventilation

SECTION EDITOR: Vinod Singh

12

CHAPTER

Basics of Mechanical Ventilation

Vinod Singh, Vitrag Shah

PHYSIOLOGY OF THE PULMONARY SYSTEM

The pulmonary system provides gas exchange. Oxygen and carbon dioxide (CO_2) are exchanged between the atmosphere and alveoli, between the alveoli and pulmonary capillary blood, and between the systemic capillary blood and all the cells of the body. Effective respiration requires gas exchange in the lungs (external respiration) and in the tissues (internal respiration). The processes for adequate oxygenation and acid-base balance are ventilation, pulmonary perfusion, and diffusion. There are four basic steps in the gas exchange process which are as follows:

1. **Ventilation:** Process of moving air.
2. **Diffusion:** Process by which alveolar air gases are moved across the alveolar-capillary membrane to the pulmonary capillary bed and vice versa.
3. **Transport of gases into circulation:** Approximately 97% of oxygen is transported in chemical combination with hemoglobin (Hgb) in the erythrocyte and 3% is carried dissolved in the plasma. PaO_2 is a measurement of the oxygen carried in the plasma.
4. **Diffusion between systemic capillary bed and body tissue cells:** Diffusion of O_2 and CO_2 in the systemic capillaries, interstitial fluid, and cells.

The use of ventilators has been recorded since the early 1800s, but modern ventilation was first used in the 1940s. The early mechanism was based on keeping the chest in a negative-pressure environment that was contained in a closed system such as the "iron lung." As technology advanced, so did the benefits. Healthcare providers were able to perform surgeries that were not possible without mechanical ventilation, and many patients who previously would not have survived recovered from infections such as pneumonia. However, there were also drawbacks. The equipment was large and difficult to use. Most ICUs were not able to handle more than four or five ventilated patients, and there was difficulty maintaining adequate ventilation. The ventilators in use today use positive pressure—the forcing of gases into the chest—instead of negative pressure. When a patient is put on a ventilator, numerous settings, including respiratory rate, fraction of inspired oxygen (FiO_2), volume or pressure control, and ventilator mode, must be selected. In addition, two adjuncts— positive end expiratory pressure (PEEP) and pressure support—are sometimes used. To efficiently care for your patient, it is important to understand each of these settings.

GOALS OF MECHANICAL VENTILATION

1. Relieve respiratory distress
2. Decrease work of breathing
3. Improve pulmonary gas exchange
4. Reverse respiratory muscle fatigue
5. Permit lung healing
6. Avoid complications.

VENTILATOR SETTINGS

1. Ventilator mode
2. Oxygen concentration
3. Tidal volume
4. Set rate
5. Inspiratory flow rate
6. Inspiration: Expiration ratio
7. Positive end expiratory pressure.

Inspired Oxygen Concentration

- Initially select high FiO_2 and adjust when obtain arterial blood gases (ABGs) after 20 minutes.
- Aim for lowest FiO_2 that will achieve PaO_2 of 60–70 mm Hg (or SpO_2 of 90%).
- PEEP may be required to achieve a decrease in FiO_2
- Oxygen toxicity:
  - Exposure to FiO_2 of 1.0 up to 24 hours does not result in a significant clinical risk, but beyond that time it is clearly toxic.
  - An FiO_2 of 0.50 is generally considered safe for several weeks if required.
  - For FiO_2 between 0.5 and 1.0, the duration of safe exposure prior to the onset of toxicity in humans is unknown.
  - When managing hypoxemic patients, there is more to fear from severe hypoxemia than the potential threat of oxygen toxicity.

Tidal Volume

1. Tidal volume during normal spontaneous breathing equals 5 mL/kg. Employment of this volume during mechanical ventilation results in atelectasis which can be avoided by using intermittent sighs.

2. Large tidal volumes of 10–15 mL/kg may produce alveolar injury.
3. Preferred tidal volume = 6–8 mL/kg
4. Remember that some volume is lost (due to compression) in the circuit.

Ventilator Rate

- On bedside chart, record both the rate set on the ventilator and the patient's total respiratory rate
  a. Intermittent mandatory ventilation (IMV)
     - Initially, set rate should be close to the patient's total rate
     - Slowly decrease set rate with patient's tolerance in order to wean
  b. Assist control
     - Back-up rate should be 2–4 breaths below spontaneous rate
     - Decreasing set rate does not decrease level of support.

Inspiratory Flow Rate

- An inspiratory flow rate (IFR) of 60 L/min achieves optimal gas exchange in most patients.
- An IFR of 100 L/min achieves better gas exchange in patients with chronic obstructive pulmonary disease (COPD), probably because the decrease if inspiration:expiration (I:E) ratio (with prolongation of expiration) allows more complete emptying of gas-trapped regions.
- An inappropriately low IFR can markedly increase the active work of breathing by a patient.

Inspiration: Expiration Ratio

- Usually 1:2
- Inverse ratio ventilation (up to 4:1).

POSITIVE END EXPIRATORY PRESSURE

Goals

- Improve oxygenation and minimize risk of oxygen toxicity of excess fluid within the lung. By recruiting collapsed alveoli, it permits inspiration to occur on the steep portion of the pressure-volume curve. These changes combined with possible redistribution of excess fluid within the lungs result in a decrease in shunt.
- Modify natural course of lung injury; however, prophylactic PEEP does not decrease the risk of acute respiratory distress syndrome (ARDS) in patients at risk.

Institution of PEEP

1. Ensure that PEEP is the only variable being altered

2. Use stepwise increments (3–5 cm H_2O)
3. Minimize interval between change and evaluation.

Optimal PEEP

- Subject of controversy.
- Do not base PaO_2 solely (as improvement in PO_2 may be accompanied by cardiovascular impairment).
- As a general rule, optimal PEEP is achieved by maximizing O_2 delivery at lowest FiO_2 setting.
- Measurements of shunt fraction and thoracic compliance have been used as a guide to optimal PEEP; these are no longer commonly employed on routine basis.

Decreasing PEEP

- Abrupt reduction in PEEP may produce severe hypoxemia that takes days to reverse.
- Need stable patient with PaO_2 >80 mm Hg and $FiO_2 \leq 0.40$ before decreasing PEEP.
- Harbor view Three-Minute Rule:
  - Measure PaO_2 and decrease PEEP by ≤5 cm H_2O
  - Obtain ABG after 3 minutes and immediately return PEEP to previous setting.
  - If PaO_2 falls by >20%, maintain PEEP at previous setting.
  - If PaO_2 falls by <20%, there is a 90% likelihood that PEEP can be successfully decreased.

Common Conditions Needing Mechanical Ventilation

- Acute lung injury (including ARDS, trauma)
- Apnea with respiratory arrest, including cases from intoxication
- Chronic obstructive pulmonary disease (COPD)
- Acute respiratory acidosis with partial pressure of carbon dioxide (pCO_2) >50 mm Hg and pH <7.25, which may be due to paralysis of the diaphragm due to Guillain-Barré syndrome, myasthenia gravis, spinal cord injury, or the effect of anesthetic and muscle relaxant drugs
- Increased work of breathing as evidenced by significant tachypnea, retractions, and other physical signs of respiratory distress
- Hypoxemia with arterial partial pressure of oxygen (PaO_2) with supplemental fraction of inspired oxygen (FiO_2) < 55 mm Hg
- Hypotension including sepsis, shock, congestive heart failure
- Neurological diseases such as muscular dystrophy amyotrophic lateral sclerosis

Modes of Ventilation

Volume Control

Traditionally, mechanical ventilation is volume controlled. This setting means the ventilator is programmed to deliver a preset volume of oxygen and air, called the tidal volume (V_T), regardless of the amount of pressure required to deliver the volume (a positive pressure alarm protects patients from dangerously high pressures).

Pressure Control

An alternative to volume control that's indicated for some patients, pressure control simply means that pressure is the endpoint rather than volume. Thus, inspiration ends when a preset pressure is reached, regardless of the volume delivered.

The advantage of this mode is that it allows the volume to change in response to intrathoracic pressure. The goal is to increase mean airway pressure by prolonging inspiration, ideally recruiting more alveoli than volume control ventilation. By limiting pressure, there is less risk of pressure-related injury.

Pressure-regulated Volume Control (PRVC)

This type of mechanical ventilation is an alternative to strict pressure control, representing an attempt to obtain the best of both volume and pressure control. PRVC adapts to changing compliance of the lungs to adjust inspiratory time and pressure to maintain a preset tidal volume.

Assist Control (AC)

In this mode, the ventilator supports every breath, whether it's initiated by the patient or the ventilator. It is similar to volume control except that the patient is allowed to breathe and trigger breaths. Because AC mode results in the higher level of positive pressure in the chest, it increases the risk of barotrauma to the lungs. Anxious patients who frequently trigger the ventilator can easily hyperventilate.

Synchronized Intermittent Mandatory Ventilation (SIMV)

In this mode, not all spontaneous breaths are assisted, leaving the patient to draw some breaths on her own. For example, if your patient's ventilator is set on SIMV mode with a respiratory rate of 10 bpm, she will receive a breath roughly once every six seconds. She can also breathe on her own in between the machine-assisted breaths.

There are several advantages to this mode for patients who can tolerate it. SIMV helps preserve the strength of the respiratory musculature, decreases the risk of hyperventilation and barotrauma, and facilitates weaning. Weaning can be done by gradually decreasing the percentage of machine-assist ventilation.

Patients who need short-term ventilation benefit most from SIMV, but the choice of mode should be an individual decision based on the patient's condition and tolerance. No one method is best for all patients.

Dual-modes of Ventilation

Combine volume and pressure targets.

Preparing for Intubation: Positioning and Bagging

Prior to intubation, a team member should be bagging (ventilating) the patient with 100% oxygen (O_2).

- Another team member should be monitoring the patient's vital signs (including pulse oximetry), ensuring IV access and overall patient status.
- The wall suction should be turned on high and a Yankeur suction device attached and ready for use (it is convenient to place this by the patient's head).
- The patient's head of the bed should be flat with the pillow removed. The patient should be lying supine in good anatomical position with the shoulders square and the head in the sniffing position (the patient's neck is flexed slightly forward and the head is extended up and back in order to open a partially obstructed upper airway). The physician will likely need the bed elevated to facilitate tube placement. He or she might ask you to place a small rolled up towel or folded blanket under the shoulders or neck; this will also help to facilitate tube placement.
- Always get good IV access, attach fluids and keep emergency drugs ready.

Monitoring during Mechanical Ventilation

Continuous electrocardiography (ECG), blood pressure, and pulse oximetry (SaO_2) are mandatory. An arterial blood gas (ABG) measurement is frequently obtained 10–15 minutes after the institution of mechanical ventilation. The measured arterial PaO_2 should verify the pulse oximetry readings and direct

Table 1: Initial ventilator settings for adult patients

	Tidal volume	*Resp rate*	*I:E Ratio*	*PEEP*	*FiO_2*
Normal lungs	8 mL/kg	12–15	1:2	5	1.0
Asthma/ COPD	6 mL/kg	10–12	1:4	5	1.0
ARDS	6 mL/kg	12–15	1:2	5–15	1.0
Hypov-olemia	8 mL/kg	12–15	1:2	0–5	1.0

Abbreviations: PEEP, positive end expiratory pressure; COPD, chronic obstructive pulmonary disease; ARDS, acute respiratory distress syndrome.

the reduction of FiO_2 to a value less than 0.5. The measured $PaCO_2$ can suggest adjustments of minute ventilation but should be interpreted in light of the patient's overall acid-base status. For example, full correction of $PaCO_2$ in a chronically hypercarbic COPD patient will lead to unopposed metabolic alkalosis.

Besides arterial blood gas measurement monitoring of end-tidal CO_2 is very helpful. The advantage of end-tidal CO_2 monitoring is that it can detect acute ventilator dysfunction such as endotracheal tube obstruction or dislodgement.

Peak inspiratory and plateau pressures should be assessed frequently, although it should be recognized that both pressures will be increased by extrapulmonary factors such as stiff chest wall or a distended abdomen. In general, however, set parameters may need to be altered to limit pressures to less than 35 cm H_2O. Expiratory tidal volume is checked initially and periodically (continuously if ventilator is capable) to ensure that the set tidal volume is delivered. Any discrepancy between delivered tidal volume and that manually selected must prompt a search for air leak such as underinflated tube cuffs, open tubing ports, or worsening pneumothorax. In patients with airway obstruction, monitor auto-PEEP.

Ventilator Troubleshooting

The differential diagnosis of the clinically deteriorating, mechanically ventilated patient is wide and includes endotracheal tube or ventilator dysfunction, improper ventilator settings, pain, anxiety, and pulmonary or extrapulmonary disease processes.

The complications most commonly encountered in the while patient is on a ventilator include hypoxia, hypotension, high-pressure alarms, and low exhaled-volume alarms.

Intubated patients who develop hemodynamic instability with respiratory compromise should immediately be disconnected from the ventilator and manually ventilated with 100% FiO_2.

One of the first diagnoses that should be considered in any hemodynamically unstable patient undergoing positive-pressure ventilation is tension pneumothorax. This is a clinical diagnosis and should be treated with needle decompression prior to obtaining a chest radiograph.

A second diagnosis to exclude, particularly in patients with asthma or COPD, is intrinsic PEEP. As discussed, intrinsic PEEP occurs as a result of incomplete exhalation, which subsequently leads to hyperinflation, increased intrathoracic pressure, decreased venous return, and decreased preload. The diagnosis of intrinsic PEEP may be made by performing an end-expiratory hold or by detecting a flow not returning to zero at end expiration.

Other diagnoses to consider are an obstructed endotracheal tube and an endotracheal tube cuff leak. In the case of endotracheal tube obstruction, attempts to manually ventilate the patient are met with a significant amount of resistance and high-pressure alarms may sound. Endotracheal tube obstruction may be caused by extrinsic compression; tube plugs with mucus, blood, or foreign bodies; tube kinks; or tube biting. Tube suctioning and adequate patient sedation are recommended after other causes of obstruction are ruled out.

Measurement of peak pressures and plateau pressures may be helpful in identifying the location of resistance, especially if graphical representation of airway pressures is available. Peak pressure, which reflects resistance to airflow, is measured by the ventilator during inspiration. High peak pressure with normal plateau pressures indicates increased resistance to flow, such as endotracheal tube obstruction or bronchospasm. An increase in both peak and plateau pressures suggest decreased lung compliance, which may be seen in disease states such as pneumonia, ARDS, pulmonary edema, and abdominal distention.

Low exhaled volume alarms are triggered by air leaks. These are most frequently secondary to ventilatory tubing disconnect from the patient's tracheal tube but will also occur in the event of balloon deflation or tracheal tube dislodgement. Tube placement, balloon inflation, and connection to the ventilator should be carefully verified.

Hypoxia after intubation may occur secondary to hypoventilation, worsening cardiac shunting, inadequate FiO_2, mainstem intubation, aspiration, tube dislodgement, or pulmonary edema. The causes of high airway pressures and low exhaled volumes described above can result in hypoxia if they cause hypoventilation. Despite the use of numerous safety precautions, cases are occasionally documented of ventilators being connected to compressed air or nitrous oxide rather than oxygen. Increasing FiO_2 and adjusting ventilatory settings to increase PEEP or respiratory rate are useful first steps after excluding equipment failure and mechanical causes of hypoxia.

Hypotension after intubation is usually attributable to diminished central venous blood return to the heart secondary to elevated intrathoracic pressures. This can be treated with fluid infusions and/or adjustment of ventilatory settings to lower intrathoracic pressure (reducing PEEP, tidal volume, and, if air trapping is suspected, respiratory rate). Hypotension may also be secondary to vasovagal reaction to intubation, rapid sequence induction, sedation, and tension.

Supportive Care

It becomes important to initiate preventative measures to decrease the incidence of the secondary complications of mechanical ventilation, such as ventilator-associated pneumonia (VAP), venous thromboembolism (VTE), and stress-related mucosal injury.

The Centers for Disease Control and Prevention published Guidelines for Preventing Health-Care Associated Pneumonia in which they recommend placing the patient in a semiupright position, with the head of the bed elevated 30–45°, in order to reduce the risk of aspiration.

Other measures such as early placement of a nasogastric tube and oral care with a soft toothbrush and chlorhexidine rinses may also be considered. Endotracheal cuff pressures should be monitored initially after intubation and every 4 hours thereafter, with goal pressures of 20–30 cm H_2O.

In patients without contraindications, unfractionated or low-molecular-weight heparin should be considered in these patients for deep venous thrombosis. As the incidence of gastric mucosal erosions has been found to be greater than 75% in ICU patients within 24 hours of admission, proton pump inhibitor, sucralfate, or histamine receptor antagonist should be considered in patients especially in high-risk patients such as those with coagulopathy, history of gastrointestinal bleeding, history of gastritis or peptic ulcer, or mechanical ventilation for more than 48 hours.

13
CHAPTER

Noninvasive Ventilation

Vinod Singh

NONINVASIVE VENTILATION

Noninvasive ventilation (NIV) refers to the delivery of mechanical ventilation to the lungs using techniques which do not require endotracheal airway. The interface that replaces the endotracheal tube are different types of masks, nasal or full face mask or a helmet. NIV can be further categorized as noninvasive positive pressure ventilation (NIPPV) or continuous airway positive pressure (CPAP). NIPPV provides inspiratory pressure support (also referred to as IPAP) usually in combination with PEEP. CPAP does not actively support ventilation but provides continuous positive pressure throughout the respiratory cycle. The term Biphasic positive airway pressure (BIPAP) is also used to refer non invasive pressure support ventilation and the acronym BIPAP is registered with respironics, a manufacturer of various noninvasive devices.

Advantages of NIV

Preserves airway defence and prevents endotracheal tube related infections like pneumonia, leading to shorter ICU stay. Easier nursing care and feeding is possible. Patient compliance is better as the patient can talk and eat orally. NIV is less costly for the patient and can be used in the ward or home.

Indications of NIV

The success of NIV depends on careful patient selection. The patient must be mentally alert enough to follow commands. Clinical situations in which it has proven to be useful include acute exacerbation of chronic obstructive pulmonary disease (COPD) or asthma, decompensated congestive heart failure (CHF) with mild-to-moderate pulmonary edema.

Reviews of the literature have shown noninvasive positive-pressure ventilation (NPPV) to be beneficial for COPD, reducing the rate of tracheal intubations and the length of stay. Recently developed clinical guidelines recommend that NIPPV be considered as an adjunct to standard medical therapy in patients with severe COPD exacerbations (pH <7.35 and relative hypercarbia). In addition, it is also recommended in patients with cardiogenic pulmonary edema and respiratory failure without shock or acute coronary syndrome requiring urgent percutaneous coronary intervention.

The use of NPPV has been less well studied in asthma, though a recent meta-analysis found that NPPV improved secondary outcomes such as number of hospital admissions, length of ICU stay, and length of hospital stay. However, the study did not demonstrate a definite benefit of NIPPV for mortality or intubation rates.

Noninvasive ventilation may be used as an adjunct to weaning to reduce the duration of mechanical ventilation and the associated complications of intubation. However extra effort is required on the part of nurses to recognize its failure so that re intubation is not delayed.

Other Indications

- Neuromuscular disorders, e.g. muscular dystrophy
- Severe obstructive sleep apnea
- Palliative therapy in terminal malignancy, interstitial lung disease.

Contraindication of NIV

- Arrest: Cardiac/respiratory, hemodynamic instability
- Non-respiratory causes of respiratory failure: gastro-intestinal bleeding, arrhythmias, etc.
- Facial trauma/airway obstruction
- Inadequate upper airway reflexes
- Increased secretions or risk of aspiration
- Recent upper airway or gastrointestinal surgery.

Interfaces

Noninvasive ventilation requires an interface that connects the patient to the ventilator or a flow generator with a CPAP valve. The selection of the interface can have a bearing on the success or failure of NIV. Complete face masks that cover both the nose and mouth are the most preferred. However nasal masks which cover only the nose offer the advantage that they allow the patient to eat or drink. They may be preferred if long-term use is intended. Other interface include the helmet more preferred in the paediatrics setting which consists of a transparent hood that covers the whole head with a neck collar.

Initiation of Noninvasive Ventilation

For NIV to be successful should be comfortable with it. Patient acceptance can be aided by prior explananation of the process to the patient. The nurse can help by holding the mask gently on the patient's face so that he/she can get used to the blast of air. Once he gets used to that the straps can be secured. One must put paddings on the places the patient feels discomfort. The patient may be allowed to take short breaks from the mask.

Monitoring

Noninvasive ventilation places great responsibility on nurses as it tends to induce a sense of complacence on the part of health care personnel. The patient should be closely monitored for respiratory and hemodynamic stability. The fall in respiratory rate as well as the heart rate is a re assuring sign. Arterial blood gases (ABG) done after suitable interval can confirm the effectiveness or otherwise of the entire process.

Detecting NIV Failure

Failure to respond to NIV within 1–2 hours is demonstrated by increasing anxiety, tachycardia and tachypnea. This is confirmed by worsening gas exchange on the ABG and pulse oximetry.

A decreasing level of consciousness, confusion or drowsiness may be an indication of urgent endotracheal intubation.

Complications

The most common complication of NIV is pressure ulcers. Tight fitting mask may produce pressure ulcers on the bridge of the nose and forehead. Air leaks may produce irritation of the eyes. Dry gas under high pressure may produce oral and nasal dryness as well as aerophagia. This may lead to gastric distension. Relatively rare complications of NIV may include gastric aspiration and hemodynamic instability. Some patients may feel claustrophobic by the mask.

Air leaks are always present, if significant can greatly compromise NIV. The machine may fail to cycle and asynchrony may result. The leak compensating mechanisms of modern ventilators are as efficient as their portable counterparts.

5 Section

Fluids and Transfusion Therapy

SECTION EDITOR: Subhash Todi

14

CHAPTER

Fluid Replacement Therapy

Mohan Maharaj, Disha Magatpalli

The total body water is on an average 60% of the total body weight, out of which nearly two-thirds is intracellular and one-thirds is extracellular.

Of the extracellular, three-fourths is interstitial fluid and one-fourths is plasma.

A correct fluid prescription needs good understanding of patient physiology and fluid composition. A wrong fluid prescription can lead to a delayed recovery, organ dysfunction and death.

DISTRIBUTION OF FLUIDS IN BODY

Fluid balance can usually be determined by proper history and thorough examination (Fig. 1).

Assess indication for fluid and remember the 5 Rs of fluid therapy while prescribing fluids:

- Resuscitation
- Routine maintenance
- Redistribution
- Replacement
- Reassessment.

Assessment

- History (intake, thirst, quantity and composition of abnormal losses and any comorbidities, including malnourishment).
- Clinical examination (pulse, blood pressure, capillary refill, jugular venous pressure, presence of pulmonary or peripheral edema and presence of postural hypotension).

Current Medications

- Clinical monitoring (National Early Warning Score (NEWS), fluid balance charts, weight).
- Laboratory investigations (trends in full blood count, urea, creatinine and electrolytes).

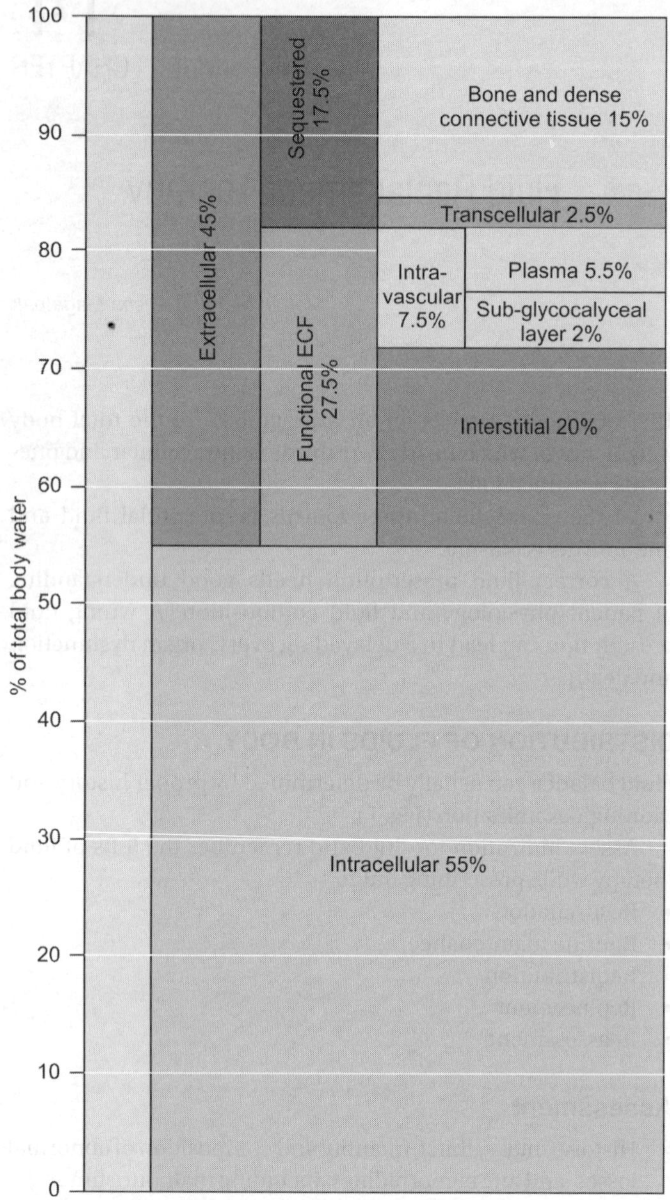

Fig. 1: Distribution of total body water

Different Phases of Fluid Resuscitation in Acute Care Setting

Salvage (in shock state): To restore vital organ perfusion—An initial fluid 'challenge' or bolus of crystalloid is recommended in doses of 500 mL in less than 15 minutes containing sodium of 130 to 154 mmol/L. Consider smaller fluid (200–300 mL in 30 minutes) in elderly, frail, and malnourished patients and with renal and cardiac impairment. Patients with intravascular fluid depletion and without shock may receive fluid at a rate of 500 mL/hour.

Optimization: To maintain the restored circulation—during the optimization phase, typically between 24 and 72 hours, the incidence of hypovolemia is substantially reduced. Smaller volumes of resuscitation fluid (5–15 mL/kg) are commonly administered during this phase triggered by episodes of oliguria or low central venous pressure or low blood pressure.

Stabilization: To prevent organ dysfunction following hemodynamic stabilization during this period unnecessary fluid administration, particularly 'maintenance' fluids and administration for drug infusions, substantially contributes to cumulative fluid balance. Using 'restrictive' fluid strategies (output ≥ intake of total fluid) will be helpful.

De-escalation: This time intrinsic hemodynamic function is restored. Try to achieve a negative fluid balance either by restricting intravenous fluid administration or by increasing fluid removal through spontaneous or induced diuresis.

Recommendations for Fluid Resuscitation in Acutely Ill-patients

Fluid resuscitation should be considered in symptomatic hypovolemia.

Fluids should be administered with the same caution that is used with any intravenous drug.

- Consider the type, dose, indications, contraindications, toxicity, and cost.
- Clearly document type of fluid to be administered and rate and volume of fluid to be administered.
- Consider all other sources of fluid and electrolyte intake, including any oral or enteral intake, intake from drugs, IV nutrition, blood and blood products.

Fluid resuscitation is a component of a complex physiological process.

- Consider fluid that is most likely to be lost. Serum electrolytes, osmolality, and acid-base status need to factored in while selecting a resuscitation fluid besides the cumulative fluid balance.
- Fluid requirements change over time in critically ill patients.
- Excessive positive fluid balance leads to interstitial edema and worse outcome.

Indicators of symptomatic hypovolemia requiring urgent fluid management

- Systolic blood pressure is less than 100 mm Hg
- Heart rate is more than 90 beats per minute
- Capillary refill time is more than 2 seconds or peripheries are cold to touch
- Respiratory rate is more than 20 breaths per minute
- Passive leg raising suggests fluid responsiveness
- Presence of postural hypotension

- Oliguria should not be used solely as a trigger or end point for fluid resuscitation.
- Avoid fluid challenge in the post-resuscitation period (≥24 hours).
- Fluid requirements decrease during the optimization and stabilization phases of resuscitation (24–96 hours).
- Fluids should be reduced or restricted during the de-escalation phase (>96 h).

Specific considerations apply to different categories of patients.

- Use isotonic, buffered salt solutions as first-line resuscitation fluids.
- Consider isotonic saline in hypovolemic, alkalotic patients and traumatic brain injury
- Use fresh whole blood or blood components in actively bleeding patients.
- Consider colloids in severely hypovolemic patients as second-line resuscitation fluids (hydroxyethyl starch is not indicated in patients with sepsis or those at risk for acute kidney injury.).
- Consider albumin during the early resuscitation of patients with severe sepsis.

Route of Fluid Administration

Peripheral IV catheters (14- to 16-gauge) are adequate for most fluid resuscitation. Maximum rate of infusion is 1 L of crystalloid in 10 to 15 minutes and 1 unit of packed RBCs in 20 minutes.

A large (e.g. 8.5 French) central venous catheter should be inserted for more rapid infusion rates and a pressure infusion device can infuse 1 unit of packed RBCs in <5 minutes. Pressure infusion device is strongly recommended in patient who are at risk of exsanguination.

Ultrasound guided placement of peripheral catheter may be needed in an oedematous patient.

Reassess Till you Reach the Goal

- Respiratory rate
- Pulse (<110/min, sinus rhythm)
- Blood pressure (MAP >75 mm Hg)
  Perfusion (capillary refill, mental state, urine output >0.5 mL/kg/hour
- ABG: pH, base excess, lactate
- Invasive monitoring
- Fluid balance chart.

Watch for Complications of Fluid Therapy

- Hypothermia
- Acid/base disturbance
- Electrolyte disturbance (hyperkalemia, hypocalcemia, hyponatremia)
- Clotting problems
- Allergic reactions
- Volume overload and pulmonary edema.

Maintenance fluids should only be used in patients unable to maintain adequate enteral hydration—consider water @ 25–30 mL/kg/day.

The 2012 Surviving Sepsis Campaign Guidelines recommend fluid resuscitation as follows:

- Crystalloids as the initial fluid of choice in the resuscitation of severe sepsis and septic shock.
- Initially target a CVP of at least 8 mm Hg (12 mm Hg in mechanically ventilated patients). Further fluid therapy is often required.
- A fluid challenge technique be applied, wherein fluid administration is continued as long as the hemodynamic improvement (e.g. arterial pressure, heart rate, urine output) continues. The rate of fluid administration be reduced substantially when cardiac filling pressures (CVP or pulmonary artery balloon-occluded pressure) increase without concurrent hemodynamic improvement.

Fluid Management in Burns

The initial resuscitation fluid in burns can be calculated by Parkland formula (Fig. 2).

- Total fluid in 1st 24 hours = 4 mL/kg BW per % burn TBSA
- Out of which half of the fluid to be given in 1st 8 hours, rest in 16 hours

Ringer lactate (RL) solution is a relatively isotonic crystalloid solution that is the key component of almost all resuscitative strategies, at least for the first 24–48 hours. It is

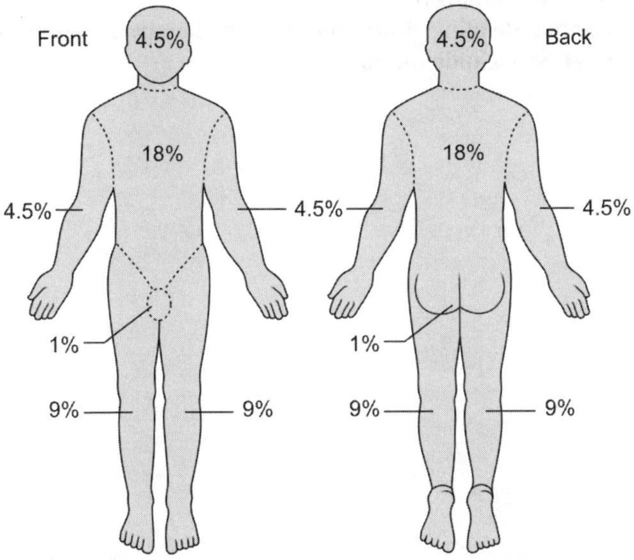

Fig. 2: Estimating the burned surface area in the adult

preferable to isotonic sodium chloride solution (i.e. normal saline) for large-volume resuscitations because of its lower sodium concentration (130 mEq/L vs 154 mEq/L) and higher pH concentration (6.5 vs 5.0). Another potential benefit of RL solution is the buffering effect of metabolized lactate on the associated metabolic acidosis. Plasmalyte is another crystalloid solution, the composition of which is more close to plasma. Plasmalyte is used in some centers as the initial crystalloid solution for large burns. However, the significant cost difference per unit, with an uncertain benefit, has limited its widespread use. Do not use colloids other than albumin.

The formula for the estimate for 5% albumin infusion is as follows:

0.5 mL/kg per percentage burn = mL albumin for 24 hours.

Modified Parkland Formula

- Initial 24 hours: RL 4 mL/kg/% burn (adults)
- Next 24 hours: Begin colloid infusion of 5% albumin 0.3–1 mL/kg/% burn/16 per hour.

Choice of Fluid and Acute Kidney Injury

The principal of fluid therapy is to maintain or restore effective intravascular volume to assure adequate tissue perfusion. Crystalloids including saline (i.e. NaCl 0.9, 0.45 or 3%), lactate-based (i.e. Hartmann's solution) or balanced (i.e. Plasma-Lyte 148) solutions are the fluids of choice for fluid resuscitation.

Hypotonic solutions are not very effective options for fluid resuscitation.

Synthetic colloids should be avoided in patients with AKI or at risk of developing AKI.

Further Reading: Intravenous fluid therapy in adults in hospital. Nice Guideline 2013.

15

CHAPTER

Blood and Blood Products

Mohan Maharaj, Disha Magatpalli

BLOOD

- A specialized fluid of the circulatory system
- Average amount of 5.6 liter/person
- Constitutes about 8% of the body weight.

Functions of Blood

- Transportation: Oxygen from the lungs to all cells of the body, carbon dioxide from the cells to the lungs. Nutrients from digestive organs to the cells.
- Regulation of body pH through buffer and amino acids.
- Maintain normal body temperature, as it contains a large volume of water which is an excellent heat absorber and coolant.
- Prevention/protection: Body fluid loss through the clotting mechanism, against toxins and foreign microbes through antibody formation.

A blood product is any component of the blood which is collected from a donor for use in a blood transfusion. Whole blood is rarely used. Blood products consist of specific processed components such as packed red blood cells, blood plasma, or platelets.

In present day practice, patients may receive a unit of packed cells or just specific components of the blood needed to treat their particular condition. Routinely four components are derived from donated blood. This approach is referred to as blood component therapy. The main blood components include: Packed cells, fresh frozen plasma (FFP), platelets and cryoprecipitate.

Erythrocytes (Red Blood Cells)

Appear as bi-concave disks, consisting of a specialized red pigment called as "Hemoglobin (Hb).

Hemoglobin form 33% of the RBC's weight and are responsible for red color of the blood and its function is to transport oxygen to the cells from the lungs and carbon dioxide from the cells to the lungs. RBC's are produced in the bone marrow by erythropoiesis and have a lifespan of 120 days. Patients who benefit most from transfusion of red blood cells include those with chronic anemia resulting from kidney failure or gastro-intestinal bleeding, and those with acute blood loss resulting from trauma.

Leukocyte depleted red blood cells require special preparation by removing leukocytes (white blood cells) by filtration shortly after donation. This is done before storage because high numbers of leukocytes remaining in a unit of RBCs during the storage process can fragment, deteriorate, and release cytokines. Leukocytes have been implicated as a cause of reactions in some transfusion recipients.

Leukocytes (White Blood Cells)

- Two subtypes: Granular and agranular
- Granular leukocytes are: Neutrophils, basophils and eosinophils.
- Agranular leukocytes are: Lymphocytes and monocytes.
- Average count varies between 4000–11000/mm.^{3}

Thrombocytes (Platelets)

- Disk-shaped anucleate cells

Prevent fluid loss by initiating a chain of reactions resulting in blood clotting.

- Have a short life span of 5–9 days.
- Average count varies between 250,000–400,000/mm^3 of blood.

PLASMA

Plasma Proteins

- Are formed in the liver and are held in the circulatory system only.
- Responsible for maintaining the colloid osmotic pressure (COP) of blood.
- Are of three subtypes: Albumin (55%), globulin (38%) and fibrinogen (7%) albumin (55%).
- Produced in the liver.
- Together with electrolytes, help in maintaining the water balance between blood and tissues and hence regulating blood volume by exerting considering osmotic pressure.
- Also provides blood with viscosity which is an important factor in the maintenance and regulation of blood pressure.

Globulin (38%): Three subtypes: Alpha (α), beta (β) and Gamma (γ): Alpha and beta globulins primarily help in transportation functions. Gamma globulins are mainly the antibodies, which provide immunity and resistance to the body against infection/toxicity.

Fibrinogen (7%): Play an essential role in the blood clotting mechanism.

Table 1: Packed red cell transfusion

Volume (mL)	*Hematocrit (L/L)*	*Hemoglobin content (g)*	*Residual plasma (mL)*	*Storage temperature*	*Shelf life*
220–340	0.5–0.7	>40	5–30	2–6°C	Up to 35 days from donation

PLATELETS

Centrifugation separates platelet rich plasma from a donated unit of whole blood raises level by approximately 5,000. This component is called platelet rich plasma (PRP).

Platelet Apheresis

Cell separator separates blood into components, retains the platelets and returns the remainder of blood to the donor (Table 2).

Table 2: Platelets from apheresis donation

Number of donors per pack	*Mean volume (mL)*	*Mean platelets (×109 per unit)*	*Anticoagulant*	*Storage*	*Shelf life*
1	199	280 (range 165–510)	Acid citrate dextrose	20–24°C with agitation	5 days

Indications

- Thrombocytopenia
- Decreased platelet production—aplastic anemia, leukemia
- Increased platelet loss—bleeding
- Increased platelet destruction = hypersplenism in cirrhosis, transfusion reaction
- Increased use or consumption = disseminated intravascular coagulopathy (DIC)
- Coagulation disorders.

FRESH FROZEN PLASMA (TABLE 3)

Prepared by freezing the plasma from 1 unit of blood at –30°C within 6 hours of donation.

Table 3: Fresh frozen plasma

Number of donor exposures per pack	*Mean volume (mL)*	*Mean Factor VIIIc (IU/mL)*	*Anticoagulant*	*Storage*	*Shelf life*
1	274	0.83 (specification >0.7)	CPD	<–25°C	36 months (24 hours at 4°C after thawing)

Indications

- Dilutional coagulopathy (i.e. massive transfusion), active bleeding, surgery or invasive procedure.
- Prothrombin time (PT) >18 seconds.
- Activated partial thromboplastin time (aPTT) > 54 seconds.
- Specific clotting factor deficiency (<25% of normal) for which other safer replacement product is not indicated.

CRYOPRECIPITATE

It was developed as a treatment for hemophilia but this use has now been replaced by factor VIII concentrate. It is rich in fibrinogen, factor VIII and von Willebrand factor. Cryoprecipitate (CRYO) is mainly used as a more concentrated source of fibrinogen than FFP.

Fresh frozen plasma from a single donor allowed to thaw at 4–8°C and removing the supernatant volume approximately 20 mL, stored at –30°C.

Table 4: Clinical use of blood products

Blood component	*Indication*	*Dose*
Platelets	Bleeding (thrombocytopenia or qualitative platelet defect)	1 unit/5 kg increases platelet 50–100 K
FFP	Coagulation disorders (replace all factors except V and VIII)	10–15 mL/kg
Cryoprecipitate	Low fibrinogen haemophilia A Von Willebrand's disease	1 unit/10 kg

ALBUMIN

There are two preparations—5% and 20%. Generally considered is preferred in renal and liver diseases inappropriate for volume resuscitation. 20% solution specially suited for nephrotic syndrome or liver disease. It is not recommended in low albumin states such as malnutrition or chronic renal/liver disease.

ADMINISTRATION OF BLOOD PRODUCTS (TABLE 4)

1. Take informed consent.
2. Cross check the identity of the patient and the blood product.
   - Verify the patients name and the hospital number both on patients wrist band and the label on the blood bag, check verbally.
   - Check blood group on the blood bag compatibility label with patients notes.
   - Note the date of expiry of the blood.
   - Look for clots or change in color, and if present discard the bag.

3. If the unit is out of controlled storage/blood bank for more than 30 minutes, then either it should be transfused immediately or marked as 'unsuitable for use' and returned.
4. IV access cannula size must be large enough to maintain an adequate flow rate for the transfusion.
5. Blood components must be transfused using an administration set with recommended filter pore size of 170–200 micron.
6. Platelets must be transfused through a new blood administration set. Platelets must not be transfused through a blood administration set which has been used for red cells, as red cell debris may trap infused platelets.
7. Remain with the patient during first 15 minutes of transfusion and monitor vital signs.
   If reaction is suspected—stop the transfusion.
   - Keep the IV line open
   - Inform doctor
   - Inform the blood bank
   - Send the blood bag with blood/urine sample of the patient to the blood bank.

16

CHAPTER

Nutritional Support in Critical Care

Subhash Todi, Mahuya Bhattacharyya

INTRODUCTION

Nutrition therapy refers to the provision of either enteral nutrition (EN) by enteral access device and/or parenteral nutrition (PN) by venous access mostly by central vein.

NUTRITIONAL ASSESSMENT

On admission to intensive care unit (ICU) all patients should be assessed for nutrition risk. Energy and protein requirements for individual patients should be calculated so also the timeline for target achievement of nutrition therapy.

- Calculation of energy need—Indirect calorimetry (IC)/ weight based calculation (25–30 kcal/kg/d).
- Calculation of protein need—weight based calculation (1.2–2 g/kg/d).
- Patients receiving hemodialysis or continuous renal replacement therapy (CRRT) should receive increased protein, up to a maximum of 2.5 g/kg/d.

ROUTES OF NUTRITIONAL SUPPORT IN CRITICAL CARE

- Enteral
- Parenteral.

Enteral Nutritional Support

Indications

Functioning gastrointestinal (GI) tract but inability to meet the needs orally, not expected to reach full oral diet in three days or unwillingness to consume nutrients.

Advantages

- Fewer complications than parenteral route
- Reduced incidence of sepsis
- Absorptive ability of GI tract maintained
- Less expensive and easy to deliver.

Contraindication of Enteral Feeding

- Absolute: Mechanical bowel obstruction
- Relative: Use of high dose of vasopressor, early stage of bowel anastomosis, paralytic ileus involving small gut.

Available Enteral Access

- Nasogastric
- Nasoduodenal
- Esophagostomy
- Gastrostomy (PEG—Percutaneous endoscopic gastrostomy)
- Jejunostomy.

Choice of access

Two main deciding factors—duration of enteral feeding and pre or postpyloric feeding.

Duration of enteral feeding

- Short-term (<6 weeks): Nasogastric or nasojejunal tube
- Long-term (>6 weeks): Gastrostomy PEG or jejunostomy.

Contraindication of gastric/prepyloric feeding

- Gastric residual volume >250 mL inspite of prokinetic
- Gastroesophageal reflux
- Risk of pulmonary aspiration (nursing in supine or prone position).

Tube Management

Tube placement

Nasogastric or nasojejunal tube is placed manually at the bedside. If nasojejunal tube cannot be placed at bedside help of fluoroscopy or endoscopy can be taken.

Contraindication/cautious placement of NG/NJ tube

- Upper gastrointestinal surgery
- Gastrointestinal bleed
- Coagulopathy
- Facial/base of skull fracture
- Esophageal varices.

Securing tube

Assessment of gut functions

- Observation of gastric tube aspirate
- Visual inspection/palpation of abdomen (tender, distended)
- Recording the frequency, nature and quantity of motions passed
- Presence/absence of bowel sounds

- Wipe and remove oil from nose
- Prepare tape in the way shown in picture
- Put tape(a) on nose, wrap wings(b) along the tube
- Secure further with another tape(c)

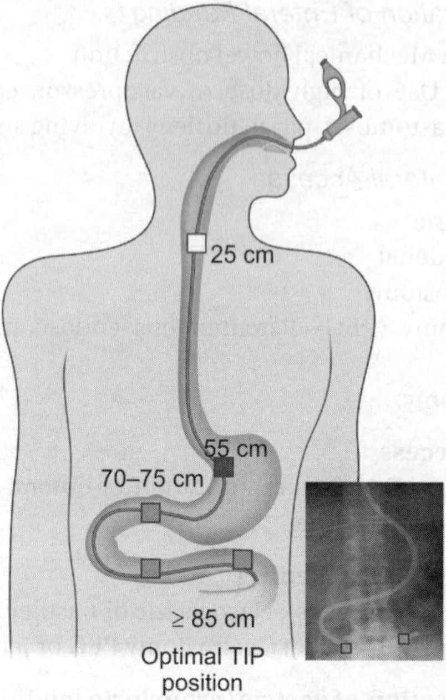

Fig. 1: Tube position inside abdomen

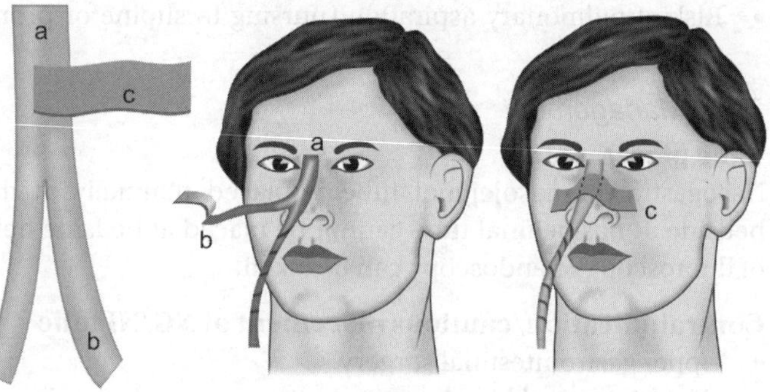

Fig. 2: Securing feeding tube with tape

Tube care

- Prevent occlusion: Flash tube with 20 mL water 4 hourly or if feeds are on hold, avoid gel or globular form or bulk forming agent, flush after medication.
- Occluded tube: Use a mixture of pancreatic enzyme, sodium bicarbonate and water—pump the liquid. If not relieved leave the solution for 2–4 hours—if still not relieved after several attempts try to insert guide wire (NJ)—if failed change the tube.

Selection of Formulas

Intensive care unit (ICU) patients should receive a standard EN formula. It may be changed only if indicated by past-medical history or any specific current medical condition.

Whole protein formulas should be used unless the patient demonstrates intolerance, or gastrointestinal complications (i.e. short bowel syndrome, pancreatitis, Crohn's disease, etc.).

Soluble fiber may be beneficial for patient receiving EN who develops diarrhea. Avoid in patients at high-risk for bowel ischemia or severe dysmotility.

Avoid calorically dense formulations for patients with hypernatremia.

Standard enteral formulations should be used in ICU patients with acute and chronic liver or kidney disease.

Patients with severe acute pancreatitis may be fed enterally by the jejunal route, by peptide-based, or nearly fat-free elemental formulation. When EN is not feasible, the use of parenteral nutrition (PN) should be considered.

For patients with a history of diabetes, lower carbohydrate content (33–40%) formula should be used.

Necessary to note osmolality of the prepared feed (isotonic is 250 to 350 mOsm/L).

Necessary to note calorie concentration (most 1 kcal/mL, but some critical care solutions such as renal resource have 2 kcal/mL).

Types

- Complete isotonic balanced liquid nutrition (e.g. Osmolite, Isocal).
- Complete balanced liquid nutrition (e.g. Ensure, Sustacal).
- High-calorie complete balanced liquid nutrition (e.g. Ensure Plus).
- High-nitrogen liquid nutrition (e.g. Magnacal, Ensure HN, Osmolite HN, Sustacal HC, Replete).
- Fiber-containing formulas (e.g. Ensure with fiber, Jevity, Sustacal with fiber).
- Partially hydrolyzed or elemental diets (e.g. Criticare HN, Impact, Vivonex).
- Specialized nutrition (e.g. Pulmocare, Glucerna SR).
- Immune-modulating formulae (formulae enriched with arginine, nucleotides and ω-3 fatty acids).

Pattern of Delivery

The delivery of feed can either be intermittent e.g. every 4 hourly by a gravity bag or it can be continuous by an infusion pump. Jejunal feeds are preferably given by continuous infusion.

General enteral feed guidelines

- Early initiation of enteral nutrition (within 24 hours) unless hemodynamically unstable.
- Correct placement of tube to be verified with X-ray upper abdomen, injection of air with auscultation over stomach, or aspiration of gastric contents.
- Continuous feeding is given via an feeding pump and intermittent feeding is given hourly.

- Start with lower volume and gradually increase by four hours as tolerated to reach the nutritional goal within 48 hours. Watch for pain, distension residual volume or passage of flatus or stool.
- Room temperature fluids (but should be at room temperature no more than 4 hours).
- Initially 0.25–0.50 strength feed should be started at slow rate; and gradually increased.
- Free water in volume equal to 0.25–0.50 volume of feeding to prevent hyperosmolality.
- Patients receiving enteral feedings should be placed in the semi-recumbent position with the HOB 30–45°, unless otherwise indicated.
- Residual volume checked every 4 hours or before next intermittent feeding; if gastric residual volume (GRV) > 200–500 mL, consider adding motility agent (IV metoclopramide or erythromycin).
- If GRV >500 mL: hold feed × 2 hours, recheck residuals after 2 hours, if >200 mL hold feed—try to find out reason—consider gastric motility agent, small bowel feeding, change elemental formula or start TPN.
- Use supplemental parenteral nutrition in patients who cannot be fed sufficiently via the enteral route.
- Immune-modulating formulae (formulae enriched with arginine, nucleotides and ω-3 fatty acids) may be used in:
  - Elective upper GI surgical patients
  - Mild sepsis (APACHE II >15).
  - Trauma
  - Acute respiratory distress syndrome (ARDS)
- Patients with a severe undernutrition and chronic catabolic state should receive EN upto 25–30 total kcal/kg BW/day.

Complications of Enteral Feeding

- Tolerance—manage GRV
- Pulmonary aspiration—patients at high-risk should receive small bowel feed
- Metabolic complications—hyperosmolar, hyperglycemic, nonketotic dehydration—Serum glucose monitored as necessary; exogenous insulin as indicated
- Nausea and vomiting, diarrhea—proper choice of feeding and slow, constant infusion, antiemetic, motility agent.
- If constipation occurs check for signs of dehydration, increase free water after bolus feeds or add a stool softener at bed time

Reasons for diarrhea

- Decreased plasma colloidal oncotic pressure (COP) caused by low serum proteins
- Bacterial contamination
- Hypertonicity
- Alteration in normal flora from antibiotics and proliferation of clostridium difficile

Parenteral Nutritional Support

Indications

- When the enteral route is contraindicated (GI disorders)
- When the enteral route is ineffective (high calorie demands)
- All patients receiving less than their targeted enteral feeding after 2 days should be considered for supplementary PN.

Routes

- Central vein for high osmolarity PN (>850 mOsmol/L)
- Peripheral vein for low osmolarity mixtures.

Types of Catheter

- Short-term: Peripheral or central venous catheter
- Long-term: Hickman, Broviac, or Groshong catheter
- If multiple-lumen catheter used, infusion through the distal lumen.

Total Parenteral Nutrition Solution

- Minimal amount of carbohydrate required is about 2 g/kg of glucose per day (concentration: peripheral 10%; central 25%).
- Enough calories in carbohydrates (or fats) for maximal protein-sparing effect.
- LCT, MCT or mixed emulsions can be administered safely at a rate of 0.7 g/kg.
- Up to 1.5 g/kg over 12 to 24 hours 30% of nonprotein calories or at least 4% to 6% of total calories should be provided by linoleic acid to prevent deficiency of essential fatty acids.
- Amino acids 1.3–1.5 g/kg ideal body weight/day in conjunction with an adequate energy supply (including essential and nonessential amino acid).
- Electrolytes: Sodium, chloride, potassium, calcium, magnesium, phosphorus.
- Buffer: Acetate or bicarbonate.
- Minerals: Iron, zinc, copper, manganese, chromium, selenium
- Multivitamins.

Possible Additions

- Insulin (sliding scale insulin still must be administered as needed)
- Heparin
- Metoclopramide (Reglan)
- H2-receptor antagonists.

Note: All additives added under laminar hood (in pharmacy department), not on nursing unit.

Guidelines

- Insertion of central venous access and its management under strict sterile technique.
- Use a dedicated line that has not been previously used for CVP measurements.

- Port (or lumen) not to be used for drawing blood samples or infusing any other fluids.
- If hanging '3-in-1' solution (also called total nutrient admixture), necessary to monitor closely for emulsion crack; solution not to be hung, if layer of fat is seen separated at top of bag.
- Use of an inline filter necessary.
- Starting rate 1200 to 2400 kcal/day and increased to desired caloric intake.
- Constant rate (volumetric pump is essential).
- Dressing changes every 48 hours.

Monitoring

- Vital signs and infusion rate at least every 4 hours (depending on the acuity of the patient's condition)
- Intake and output
- Weight daily
- Serum glucose q6 hours or early if needed
- Catheter site check.

Complications

- Infection and sepsis: Use strict sterile dressing change technique, monitor for fever and other signs of infection.
- Hyperglycemia: Decrease rate of infusion, administer insulin therapy, monitor serum glucose levels.
- Hypoglycemia: This usually occurs with interruption of TPN infusion (e.g. catheter occlusion or accidental removal).

Assessing nutritional delivery

Prescription required calorie **Required protein**

ICU day/date	*EN/PN (detail of name of nutrition with amount/ volume)*	*Delivered calorie/ deficit*	*Delivered protein/deficit*	*Suggestion from dietitian team*

FURTHER READING

1. Development of evidence-based guidelines and critical care nurses' knowledge of enteral feeding. Crit Care Nurse. 2007;27(4): 17-22.
2. Guidelines for the Provision and Assessment of Nutrition Support Therapy in the Adult Critically Ill Patient: Society of Critical Care Medicine (SCCM) and American Society for Parenteral and Enteral Nutrition (ASPEN) J Parenter Enteral Nutr. 2016;40(2):159-211.

6

Section

Infection

SECTION EDITOR: Rajesh Mohan Shetty

17

CHAPTER

Infection Control and the ICU Bundles

Rajesh Mohan Shetty, Sharanappa

INTRODUCTION

The majority of patients admitted to intensive care unit (ICU) will receive treatment for infection at some time. Around a third will develop a nosocomial infection. Nosocomial infections are defined as infections that occur at least 48 hours after a patient is admitted to the hospital without proof of being sick beforehand. Infections that occur up to 3 days after being discharged from the hospital, or infections that occur within 30 days of a surgical procedure are also included in the definition. Rates of health-care associated infections in ICU are 3–5 times higher than that in general ward patients. In developed countries, it is estimated that between 5 and 10% of the hospitalized patients will develop hospital aquired infection. In developing countries, this proportion has been estimated to be around 25%.

Most of the nosocomial infections are caused by resistant strains of microbes. For example, one strain of *Staphylococcus aureus* has evolved into methicillin-resistant *Staphylococcus aureus*, known by the acronym MRSA. Other examples of resistant pathogens are vancomycin-resistant enterococci (VRE) and azole-resistant *Candida* species. The problem of resistant pathogens such as these came about because of the inadequate or excessive use of antibiotics and antimicrobials. These pathogens are extremely adaptive to challenges of antimicrobial therapy. When inappropriate or incomplete antibiotic course is taken the bacteria left behind that were able to resist the drug will multiply, bringing with it its resistance to the antibiotic. When it spreads to other people, they cannot be treated with the original drug, so they are prescribed a different drug, which is exactly what happened with the *S. aureus* bacteria.

Intensive care unit patients are at increased risk of nosocomial infections. This increased risk is associated with several factors, some of them are mentioned below:

- The severity of the patient's illness and underlying conditions.
- The exposure to multiple invasive devices and procedures.

- Increased patient contact with health-care personnel.
- A longer ICU stay which prolongs the risk of exposure.
- Space limitations that increase the risk of contaminating equipment.

In order to protect patients, it is necessary for a critical care nurse to become familiar with nosocomial infections. Knowing how the infections came to be and what is being done to treat them can also help health care providers. Since patients in the ICU are likely to have multiple devices for treating or monitoring their care, it is not surprising that the most common nosocomial infections are pneumonia (endotracheal tubes), urinary tract infections (urinary catheters) and catheter-related bloodstream infections. Bloodstream infections (BSI) is the most common hospital acquired infection. Most blood-stream infections are secondary to an infection at another site. Approximately 39 per 1000 patients in English ICUs develop device-related bacteremia, with the vast majority of these being due to central venous catheters. Urinary tract infection (UTI) is the most common hospital-acquired infections related to the use of indwelling catheters or instrumentation. Among patient with a UTI, 1 to 2% may actually develop bacteremia. Ventilator-associated pneumonia has mortality rates of 20–50%.

OBJECTIVES

The primary aim of the Infection Control Program is to prevent or minimize the potential for nosocomial infections in patients as well as in staff by breaking the chain of transmission. There are several sources of cross-infection in the ICU, some of them are mentioned below:

- Hands of staff and attendants
- Assisted ventilation equipments
- Suction and drainage bottles
- IV lines central and peripheral
- Urinary catheters
- Wounds and wound dressings
- Disinfectant containers
- Dressing trolleys (on which disinfectants jars/bottles are stored).

Local antibiotic policies should be developed in collaboration with clinicians, microbiologists and pharmacists and be regularly reveiwed. They are based on the nature of the local patient population and must reflect the types and susceptibility patterns of pathogens circulating within the ICU, the hospital and the local community. Empiric antibiotic therapy should be started after appropriate cultures are taken. Therapy should be adjusted to the narrowest spectrum effective antimicrobial based on culture results, and antibioitics should be stopped as soon as there is cure or if no evidence of infection is found.

Four major areas of infection control program are:

1. Standard precautions, including hand hygiene
2. Isolation precautions
3. Environmental cleaning
4. Surveillance.

STANDARD PRECAUTIONS

Standard precaution are a set of infection control practices used to prevent transmission of diseases that can be acquired by contact with blood or other body fluids through nonintact skin and mucous membranes. These measures are to be used by all critical care nurses when providing care to all individuals, whether or not they appear infectious or symptomatic.

Hand Hygiene

Hand hygiene refers to either handwashing with soap and water or the use of alcohol-based gels or foams that do not require the use of water. Hand hygiene is the single most important measure to reduce transmission of microorganisms from one person to another or one site to another on the same patient. However compliance rates of ICU handwashing procedures average 30–40%. When hands are visibly dirty or visibly soiled with blood or other body fluids, hand should be washed with either antimicrobial or non-antimicrobial soap. If hands are not visibly soiled, an alcohol-based hand rub can be used to clean the hands. Alcohol-based antiseptic hand rubs are highly effective and quicker to use and is shown to increase the compliance compared to hand wash. Handwashing should be used in patients with actual or suspected infection by diarrheal pathogens such as Norovirus and the spores of *Clostridium difficile* as hand rubs are ineffective for these pathogens.

Hands should be decontaminated before:

- Direct contact with patients
- Donning sterile gloves before sterile procedures
- Moving from a contaminated-body site to a clean-body site during patient care
- Eating

Hands should be decontaminated after:

- Contact with a patient's intact skin
- Contact with body fluids or excretions, mucous membranes, nonintact skin, and wound dressings, inanimate objects (including medical equipment) in the immediate vicinity of the patient
- Removing gloves
- Using a restroom.

Personal Protective Equipment

Appropriate use of aprons, gowns, gloves, protective eye-wear and face masks protects staff and prevents transmission of microorganisms to patients.

Gloves

Gloves (clean, nonsterile gloves are adequate) should be worn when touching blood, body fluids, secretions, excretions, and contaminated items. Clean gloves should be used just before touching mucous membranes and nonintact skin. Gloves need to be changed between tasks and procedures on the same patient after contact with material that may contain a high concentration of microorganisms. Gloves should be removed promptly after use, before touching noncontaminated items and surfaces, and before going to another patient, and hands washed immediately to avoid transfer of microorganisms to other patients or environments.

Mask, Eye Protection, Face Shield

Wear a mask and eye protection or a face shield to protect mucous membranes of the eyes, nose, and mouth during procedures and patient-care activities that are likely to generate splashes or sprays of blood, body fluids, secretions, and excretions.

Gown

Gown (a clean, nonsterile gown is adequate) protects skin and prevents soiling of clothing during procedures and patient-care activities that are likely to generate splashes or sprays of blood, body fluids, secretions, or excretions. Remove a soiled gown as promptly as possible and wash hands to avoid transfer of microorganisms to other patients or environments.

Patient-care Equipment

Used patient-care equipment soiled with blood, body fluids, secretions, and excretions should be handled in a manner that prevents skin and mucous membrane exposures, contamination of clothing, and transfer of microorganisms to other patients and environments. Ensure that reusable equipment is not used for the care of another patient until it has been cleaned and reprocessed appropriately. Single-use items should be discarded properly.

Environmental Control

Hospital should have adequate procedures for the routine care, cleaning, and disinfection of environmental surfaces, beds, bedrails, bedside equipment, and other frequently touched surfaces.

Linen

Used linen soiled with blood, body fluids, secretions, and excretions should be handled, transported and processed in a manner that prevents skin and mucous membrane exposures and contamination of clothing and that avoids transfer of microorganisms to other patients and environments.

Needle Stick and Sharp Injury Prevention

Safe handling of needles and other sharp devices are components of standard precautions that are implemented to prevent health care worker exposure to blood-borne pathogens.

- Used needles should be discarded immediately after use and not recapped, bent, cut, removed from the syringe or tube holder, or otherwise manipulated.
- Any used needles, lancets, or other contaminated sharps should be placed in a leak-proof, puncture-resistant sharps container that is labeled with a biohazard label.
- Sharps containers should not be overfilled. It should be discarded after it is two-thirds full or when contents are at the "full" line indicated on the container.

ISOLATION PRECAUTIONS

In addition to standard precautions, the following should be observed in those patients known or suspected to have airborne, contact or droplet infections

Contact Precautions

Microorganisms can be transmitted to patients via contact between the patient and a healthcare worker, or by contact between the patient and a contaminated object (such as clothing, inadequately disinfected endoscopes or other medical equipment). Examples include parainfluenza virus infection, respiratory syncytial virus infection, varicella (chickenpox), herpes zoster, hepatitis A and rotavirus infections.

Ideally, the patients who require contact precautions should either be in a private room or cohorted with patients who have the same active infection or are colonized with the same pathogen. Healthcare workers should wear nonsterile gloves for all patient contact. Gowns are required if there is likely to be substantial direct contact with the patient or any infective material. Medical equipment should idealy be dedicated to single patient use when possible.

Droplet Precautions

Microorganisms are also transmitted by droplets (large particles >5 μm in size) generated during coughing, sneezing and talking, or a short-distance traveling, for example, influenza virus, *Bordetella pertussis, Hemophilus influenzae, Neisseria meningitidis, Mycoplasma pneumoniae,* Severe acute respiratory syndrome-associated coronavirus, Group A *Streptococcus,* adenovirus and rhinovirus. Because droplets remain suspended in the air for limited periods, exposure of less than 3 feet is usally required for human-to-human transmission of droplet borne pathogens. However, droplets can occasionally be transmitted up to 6 feet from the source patients.

Healthcare workers within 6 to 10 feet of patients on droplet precautions should wear a facemask. The doors of the rooms used to these patients may remain open, in contrast to airborne precautions.

Airborne Precautions

Airborne droplets nuclei are particles of respiratory secretions smaller than 5 µm. Disease-causing microorganisms may be suspended in the air as small particles, aerosols, or dust and remain infective over time and distance, for example, *Mycobacterium tuberculosis*, varicella zoster virus (chickenpox), herpes zoster (shingles), rubella virus and measles.

Patients placed on airborne isolation precautions should be placed in an airborne infection isolation room. This should be a private room with negative air pressure and a minimum of 6 to 12 air changes per hour. Doors to the isolation rooms must remain closed, and all persons entering must wear a respirator with a filtering capacity of 95% (e.g., disposable N-95 respirator mask) that allows a tight seal over the nose and mouth. If patients in respiratory isloation require transport outside their isolation rooms for medical procedures, they should wear surgical mask that cover their mouths and noses during transport. It is preferable to carry out these procedures when the waiting areas are less crowded.

Patient Bathing

Patient bathing with chlorhexidine gluconate, an antiseptic solution with broad spectrum activity against many organisms has been demonstrated to reduce the rate of hospital aquired bloodstream infections and the risk of colonization with drug-resistant organisms among patients in intensive care units and bone marrow transplant units.

ENVIRONMENTAL CLEANING

Environmental cleaning, disinfection and sterilization are basic and important measures used to prevent or reduce infections in the hospital environment.

Cleaning

Cleaning is the removal of all foreign material (e.g. soil, organic material) from objects. It is normally accomplished with water, mechanical action and detergents or enzymatic products. Meticulous physical cleaning must always precede disinfection and sterilization procedures.

Disinfection

Disinfection describes a process that eliminates many or all pathogenic microorganisms from inanimate objects, except for bacterial spores. Disinfection is usually accomplished by the use of liquid chemicals.

Sterilization

Sterilization is the complete elimination of all forms of microbial life including spores. Steam sterilization remains the most widely used technique.

SURVEILLANCE

Effective surveillance involves counting cases, calculating rates of various infections and reporting the data in an appropriate way to personnel involved in patient care.

INTENSIVE CARE UNIT BUNDLES

The Institute of Healthcare Improvement developed the concept of bundles. A "bundle" is a group of evidence-based care components for a given disease that, when executed together, may result in better outcomes than if implemented individually. Bundles to prevent ventilator-associated pneumonia (VAP), central line-associated bloodstream infections (CLABSI) and sepsis have been shown to be powerful stimuli for instituting multiple interventions to successfully prevent infection.

Ventilator-associated Pneumonia Bundle

Reducing mortality due to VAP requires an organized process like ventilator bundle that guarantees early recognition of pneumonia and consistent application of the best evidence-based practices.

The key elements of the ventilator-associated pneumonia bundle are:

- Head of bed (HOB) elevated to 30–45°
- Deep venous thrombosis (DVT) prophylaxis
- Peptic ulcer disease prophylaxis
- Daily sedative interruption and daily assessment of readiness to extubate
- Daily oral care with chlorhexidine.

Head of Bed Elevation

Elevation of the head of the bed has been correlated with reduction in the rate of ventilator-associated pneumonia. The recommended elevation is 30 to 45 degree. Importance of elevation is that it reduces potential for aspiration. Including this intervention on nursing flow sheets and as a topic at multidisciplinary rounds, on order sets for initiation and weaning of mechanical ventilation, delivery of tube feedings, and provision of oral care may increase the compliance.

Deep Vein Thrombosis

Empowering pharmacy to review orders for patients in the ICU to ensure that some form of deep venous prophylaxis is in place at all times on ICU patients may be useful.

Gastrointestinal Prophylaxis

Aspiration causes either pneumonitis or pneumonia and can be prevented. The effects of aspirating acidic contents may be worse than those with a higher pH. Increasing the pH of gastric contents may protect against a greater pulmonary inflammatory response to aspiration of gastrointestinal (GI) contents.

Daily Sedative Interruptions and Daily Assessment of Readiness to Extubate

Daily sedative interruptions and assessing the patient's readiness to extubate has been correlated with reduction in the rate of ventilator-acquired pneumonia. Care should be taken to prevent self-extubation by increased monitoring and vigilance during the trial.

Daily Oral Care with Chlorhexidine

Studies have shown that oral decontamination of mechanically ventilated adults using chlorhexidine is associated with a lower risk of ventilator associated pneumonia. Dental plaques develops in patients that are mechanically ventilated because of the lack of mechanical chewing and the absence of saliva. Dental plaque can be a significant reservoir for potential respiratory pathogens that cause ventilator-associated pneumonia. Chlorhexidine antiseptic has been approved as an inhibitor of dental plaque formation and gingivitis. The US Food and Drug Administration recommends 0.12% oral chlorhexidine for use as mouth rinse.

CENTRAL LINE BUNDLE

Key elements of central line bundle are:

- Hand hygiene
- Maximal barrier precautions upon insertion
- Chlorhexidine skin antisepsis
- Optimal catheter site selection
- Daily review of line necessity with prompt removal of unnecessary lines.

Hand Hygiene

Empowering nurses to enforce by use of a central line checklist to be sure all processes related to central line placement are executed for each line placement is recommended. It is advisable to keep soap/alcohol-based hand washing dispensers prominently placed and make universal precautions equipment, such as gloves, only available near hand sanitation equipment. Creating an environment where reminding each other about hand washing increases compliance rate.

Maximal Barrier Precautions Upon Insertion

Maximal barrier precautions should be part of checklist for central line placement. Equipment should be ready stocked in a cart for central line placement to avoid the difficulty of finding necessary equipment to institute maximal barrier precautions.

Chlorhexidine Skin Antisepsis

Incidence of bloodstream infections is significantly reduced in patients with central vascular lines who receive chlorhexidine gluconate versus povidone-iodine for insertion-site disinfection. Solution should dry completely before an attempted line insertion.

Optimal Catheter Site Selection

Insertion of the line into a subclavian site appears to be associated with lower rates of infection than femoral or internal jugular sites, and should be used unless medically contraindicated.

Daily Review of Line Necessity with Prompt Removal of Unnecessary Lines

Assessment for removal of central lines can be part of daily goal sheets. Central lines should not be replaced routinely but on evidence of infection, however any unnecessary lines should be removed without delay. Recording time and date of line placement can help record keeping purposes and evaluation by staff to aid in decision-making.

CATHETER-ASSOCIATED URINARY TRACT INFECTION BUNDLE

Catheter-associated urinary tract infection (CAUTI) care bundle aims to reduce the incidence of urinary tract infection. Components of CAUTI bundle include:

- Insert catheters only for appropriate indications
- Leave catheters in place only as long as needed
- Ensure that only properly trained persons insert and maintain catheters
- Insert catheters using aseptic technique and sterile equipment
- Following aseptic insertion, maintain a closed drainage system
- Maintain unobstructed urine flow
- Hand hygiene and standard (or appropriate isolation) precautions.

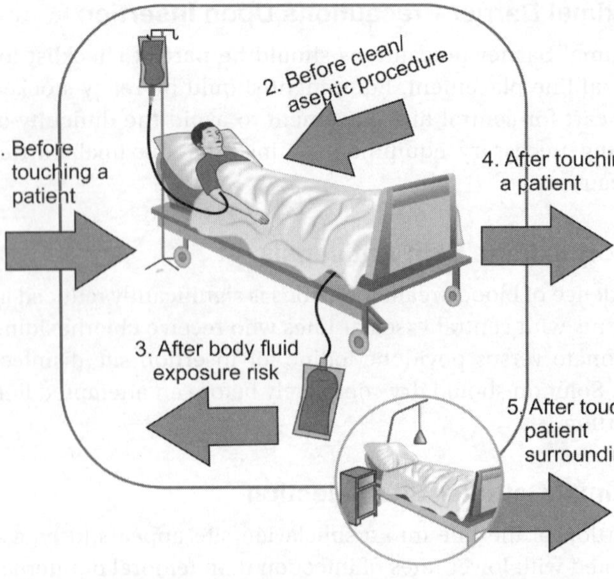

Fig. 1: World Heath Organization's five moments for hand hygiene

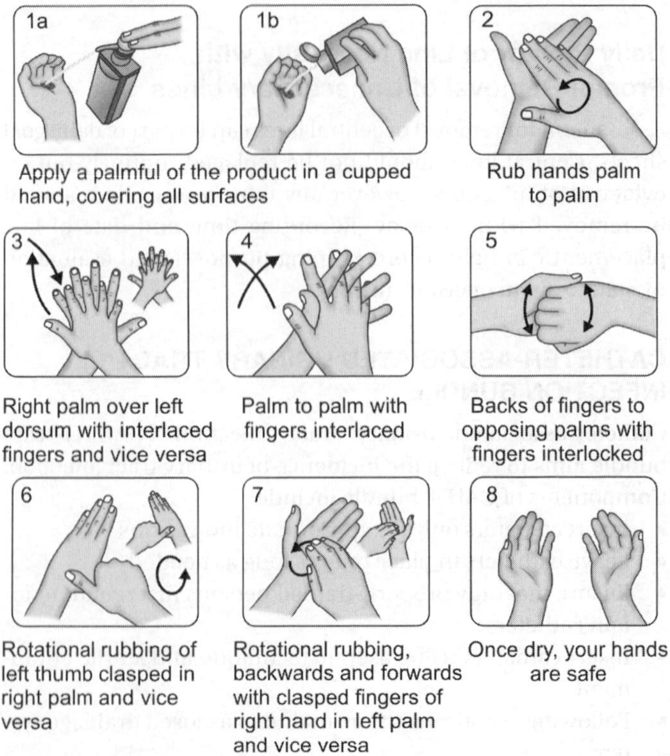

Fig. 2: Procedure for hand wash

SEPSIS BUNDLE

Sepsis bundle forms the core of the sepsis improvement efforts recommended by the Surviving Sepsis Campaign. It is divided into 3 and 6-hour bundle.

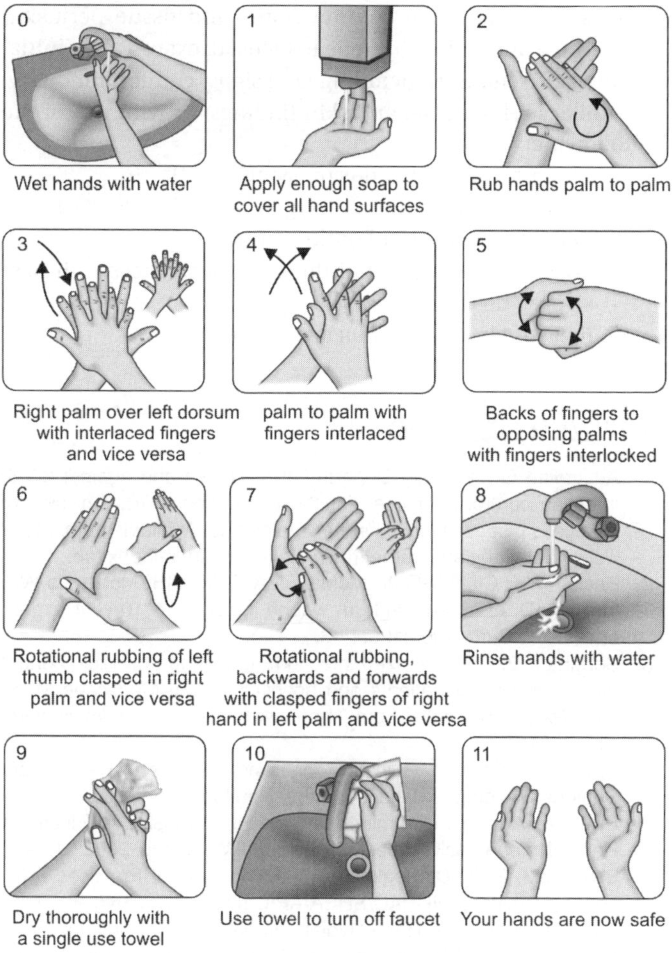

Fig. 3: Procedure for washing hands with soap and water

To be Completed within 3 Hours of Time of Presentation

- Measure lactate level
- Obtain blood cultures prior to administration of antibiotics
- Administer broad spectrum antibiotics
- Administer 30 mL/kg crystalloid for hypotension or lactate ≥4 mmol/L.

To be Completed within 6 Hours of Time of Presentation

- Apply vasopressors (for hypotension that does not respond to initial fluid resuscitation) to maintain a mean arterial pressure (MAP) ≥65 mm Hg
- In the event of persistent hypotension after initial fluid administration (MAP < 65 mm Hg) or if initial lactate was ≥4 mmol/L, reassess volume status and tissue perfusion

- Reassessment of the volume status and tissue perfusion can be done either by repeat focused exam (after initial fluid resuscitation) including vital signs, cardiopulmonary, capillary refill, pulse, and skin findings, or with two of the following:
  - Measure central venous pressure (CVP)
  - Measure central venous oxygen saturation ($ScvO_2$)
  - Bedside cardiovascular ultrasound
  - Dynamic assessment of fluid responsiveness with passive leg raise or fluid challenge
- Re-measure lactate if initial lactate elevated

FURTHER READING

1. Australian Government Department of Health and ageing; 2008. Infection control guidelines for the prevention of transmission of infectious diseases in the health care setting. Available from: http://www.health.gov.au/internet/main/./icg-guidelines-index.htm.
2. Becker WK, Cioffi WG Jr, McManus AT, Kim SH, McManus WF, Mason AD, et al. Fungal burn wound infection. A 10-year experience. Arch Surg. 1991;126:44-8.
3. Boughton B. Computerized infection monitoring and rapid control measures benefit patients and hospitals. From Medscape Medical News. Available from: http://www.medscape.com/viewarticle/725013.
4. Boyce JM, Pittet D. Guideline for Hand Hygiene in Health-Care Settings: recommendations of the Healthcare Infection Control Practices Advisory Committee and the HICPAC/SHEA/APIC/IDSA Hand Hygiene Task Force. Morbid Mortal Wkly Rep. 2002;51:1-45.
5. Boyce JM, Pittet D. Healthcare Infection Control Practices Advisory Committee; HICPAC/SHEA/APIC/IDSA Hand Hygiene Task Force. Guideline for Hand Hygiene in Health-Care Settings. Recommendations of the Healthcare Infection Control Practices Advisory Committee and the HICPAC/SHEA/APIC/IDSA Hand Hygiene Task Force. Society for Healthcare Epidemiology of America/Association for Professionals in Infection Control/Infectious Diseases Society of America. [Last accessed date March 10, 2014]. Available at http://www.cdc.gov/mmwr/pdf/rr/rr5116.pdf.
6. Burke JF, Quinby WC, Bondoc CC, Sheehy EM, Moreno HC. The contribution of a bacterially isolated environment to the prevention of infection in seriously burned patients. Ann Surg. 1977;186:377-87.
7. Centers for Disease Control and Prevention (CDC). Monitoring hospital-acquired infections to promote patient safety—United States, 1990-1999. MMWR Morb Mortal Wkly Rep. 2000;49:149-53.
8. Centers for Disease Control and Prevention, Infectious Disease Society of America, American Society of Blood and Marrow Transplantation. Guidelines for preventing opportunistic infections among hematopoietic stem cell transplant recipients. MMWR Recomm Rep. 2000;49:1-125. CE1.
9. Chastre J, Luyt CE. Ventilator-associated pneumonia. In: Mason RJ, Broaddus VC, Martin TR, et al. (Eds). Murray& Nadel's Textbook of Respiratory Medicine. 5th ed. chap 33. Philadelphia, PA: Elsevier Saunders; 2010.

10. Circulation for disinfection and sterilization in healthcare facilities. 2008. Available from:http://www.cdc.gov/hicpac/pdf/guidelines/Disinfection_Nov_2008.pdf.
11. Coffin SE, Klompas M, Classen D, Arias KM, Podgorny K, Anderson DJ, et al. Strategies to prevent ventilator-associated pneumonia in acute care hospitals. Infect Control Hosp Epidemiol. 2008;29(Suppl 1):S31-40.
12. Coffin SE, Zaoutis TE. Infection control, hospital epidemiology, and patient safety. Infect Dis Clin North Am. 2005;19:647-65.
13. Dellit TH, Owens RC, McGowan JE Jr, Gerding DN, Weinstein RA, Burke JP, et al. Infectious Diseases Society of America and the Society for Healthcare Epidemiology of America guidelines for developing an institutional program to enhance antimicrobial stewardship. Clin Infect Dis. 2007;44:159-77.
14. Department of Health U.K; 2005. ICNA Audit Tools for Monitoring ICNA Audit Tools for Monitoring Infection Control Guidelines within the Community Setting; pp. 1–48. Available at:http://www.ips.uk.net/icna/Admin/uploads/AuditTools2005.pdf.
15. Do AN, Ray BJ, Banerjee SN, Illian AF, Barnett BJ, Pham MH, et al. Bloodstream infection associated with needleless device use and the importance of infection-control practices in the home health care setting. J Infect Dis. 1999;179:442-8.
16. Drew RH. Antimicrobial stewardship programs: How to start and steer a successful program. J Manag Care Pharm. 2009;15:S18-23.
17. Dykewicz DA, Jaffe H, Spira T, et al. Guidelines for preventing opportunistic infections among hematopoietic stem cell transplant recipients: recommendations of CDC, the Infectious Disease Society of America, and the American Society of Blood and Marrow Transplantation. [Last accessed date March 10, 2014];MMWR Morb Mortal Wkly Rep. 2000 49:1-128.
18. Edmond MB, Wenzel RP. Organization for infection control. In: Mandel GL, Bennet JE, Dolin R (Eds). Principles and practice of infectious diseases. 5th ed. Philadelphia: Churchill Livingston; 2009. pp. 2988-95.
19. Edwards JR, Peterson KD, Mu Y, Banerjee S, Allen-Bridson K, Morrell G, et al. National Healthcare Safety Network (NHSN) report: Data summary for 2006 through 2008, issued December 2009. Am J Infect Control. 2009;37:783-805.
20. Erol S, Altoparlak U, Akcay MN, Celebi F, Parlak M. Changes of microbial flora and wound colonization in burned patients. Burns. 2004;30:357-61.
21. Ferdinande P. Recommendations on minimal requirements for Intensive Care Departments. Members of the Task Force of the European Society of Intensive Care Medicine. Intensive Care Med. 1997;23:226-32.
22. Fishman N. Antimicrobial stewardship. Am J Med. 2006;119(6 Suppl 1):*S53-61.*
23. French GL, Otter JA, Shannon KP, Adams NM, Watling D, Parks MJ. Tackling contamination of the hospital environment by methicillin-resistant Staphylococcus aureus (MRSA): a comparison between conventional terminal cleaning and hydrogen peroxide vapour decontamination. J Hosp Infect. 2004;57:31-7.
24. Goldmann DA, Pier GB. Pathogenesis of infections related to intravascular catheterization. Clin Microbiol Rev. 1993;6:176-92.
25. Grant PS. "The role of the infection control professional in the intensive care unit." Critical Care Nursing Quarterly 24.2 (2001): 1-12. CINAHL Plus with Full Text. EBSCO. Web. 21 Feb. 2011.

26. Green M, Avery R, Preiksaitis J. Guidelines for the prevention and management of infectious complications of solid organ transplantation. (57-109).Am J Transplant. 2004;4(Suppl 10):10-7. 160-3.
27. Guideline for isolation precautions: Preventing transmission of infectious agents in healthcare settings. 2014. Mar 10, Available from: http://www.cdc.gov/hicpac/pdf/isolation/Isolation2007.pdf.
28. Guidelines for environmental infection control in health care facilities. Available from:http://www.cdc.gov/hicpac/pdf/guidelines/eic_in_HCF_03.pdf.
29. Guidelines for prevention of catheter-associated urinary tract infections. Available fromhttp://www.cdc.gov/hicpac/pdf/CAUTI/CAUTIguideline2009final.pdf.
30. Guidelines for the prevention of intravascular catheter-related infections. Available fromhttp://www.cdc.gov/hicpac/pdf/guidelines/bsi-guidelines-2011.pdf.
31. Haley RW, Culver DH, White JW, Morgan WM, Emori TG, Munn VP, et al. The efficacy of infection surveillance and control programs in preventing nosocomial infections in US hospitals. Am J Epidemiol.1985;121:182-205.
32. Hargreaves S. UK team adopts unique approach to hospital infection control. The Lancet. 2008;8(12):747.
33. Infection control program quality monitoring indicators. Vs 2. NSW Department of Health. 2005. Available at www.health.nsw.gov.au/pubs/2005/pdf/infection_ctrl_manual.pdf.
34. Kates SG, McGinley KJ, Larson EL, Leyden JJ. Indigenous multiresistant bacteria from flowers in hospital and nonhospital environments. Am J Infect Control. 1991;19:156-61.
35. Lautenbach E. Expanding the universe of methicillin-resistant staphylococcus aureus prevention. Ann Intern Med. 2008;148:474-6.
36. Lesseva M. Central venous catheter-related bacteraemia in burn patients. Scand J Infect Dis.1998;30:585-9.
37. Linden PK. Approach to the immunocompromised host with infection in the intensive care unit. Infect Dis Clin North Am. 2009;23:535-56.
38. Lorente L, Blot S, Rello J. Evidence on measures for the prevention of ventilator-associated pneumonia. Eur Respir J. 2007;30:1193-207.
39. Maselli DJ, Restrepo MI. Strategies in the prevention of ventilator-associated pneumonia. Ther Adv Respir Dis. 2011;5:131-41.
40. McManus AT, McManus WF, Mason AD Jr, Aitcheson AR, Pruitt BA Jr. Microbial colonization in a new intensive care burn unit. A prospective cohort study. Arch Surg. 1985;120:217-23.
41. Mermel LA, Allon M, Bouza E, Craven DE, Flynn P, O'Grady NP, et al. Clinical practice guidelines for the diagnosis and management of intravascular catheter-related infection: 2009 Update by the Infectious Diseases Society of America. Clin Infect Dis. 2009; 49:1-45.
42. Mody L, McNeil SA, Sun R, Bradley SE, Kauffman CA. Introduction of a waterless alcohol-based hand rub in a long-term-care facility. Infect Control Hosp Epidemiol. 2003;24:165-71.
43. Mody L. Infection control issues in older adults. Clin Geriatr Med. 2007;23:499-514.
44. Muto CA, Jernigan JA, Ostrowsky BE, Richet HM, Jarvis WR, Boyce JM, et al. SHEA guideline for preventing nosocomial transmission of multidrug-resistant strains of Staphylococcus aureus and Enterococcus. Infect Control Hosp Epidemiol. 2003;24:362-86.
45. Nishimura S, Kagehira M, Kono F, Nishimura M, Taenaka N. Handwashing before entering the intensive care unit: What we learned from continuous video-camera surveillance. [Last accessed date March 10, 2014];Am J Infect Control. 1999 27:367-9.

46. Perz JF, Thompson ND, Schaefer MK, Patel PR. US outbreak investigations highlight the need for safe injection practices and basic infection control; Clin Liver Dis. 201014:137-51.
47. Pittet D, Allegranzi B, Sax H, Bertinato L, Concia E, Cookson B, et al. Considerations for a WHO European strategy on health-care-associated infection, surveillance, and control. Lancet Infect Dis. 2005;5:242-50.
48. Pittet D. Hand hygiene: improved standards and practice for hospital care. Curr Opin Infect Dis. 2003;16:327-35.
49. Plowman R, Graves N, Griffin M, Roberts JA, Swan AV, Cookson B, et al. The socioeconomic burden of hospital acquired infection. London Public health laboratory service and the London school of hygiene and tropical Medicine. 1999.
50. Raghunath D. Emerging antibiotic resistance in bacteria with special reference to India. J Biosci. 2008;33:593-603.
51. Ray B, Samaddar DP, Todi SK, Ramakrishnan N, John G, Ramasubban S. Quality indicators for ICU: ISCCM guidelines for ICUs in India. Indian J Crit Care Med. 2009;13(4):173-206.
52. Recommendations for preventing transmission of infections among chronic hemodialysis patients.MMWR Recomm Rep. 2001;50:1-43.
53. Review of outcomes data analysis HLTIN403B-Implement and monitor infection control policies and procedures. Available from: http://www.riskresponse.com. au/training/units-of-competency/hlt07-health/hltin403b-implement-and-mon*itor-infection-contro*l-po*licies-and* -procedures.
54. Rhodes A, Phillips GS, et al. Surviving Sepsis Campaign: association between performance metrics a*nd outcomes in a 7.5* –year study. Intensive Care Med. 2014;40:1623-33.
55. Shah RC, Shah P. Antimicrobial stewardship in institutions and office practices. Indian J Pediatr. 2008;75:815-20.
56. Starling B. Postnote July 2005 Number 247 Infection control in healthcare settings. [Last accessed date March 10, 2014]. Available from: http://www.parliamentuk/parliamentary_offices/post/pubs2005.cfm.
57. Wenzel RP. The Lowbury Lecture. The economics of nosocomial infections. J Hosp Infect. 1995;31:79-87.
58. WHO guidelines on hand hygiene in health care: A summary. 2014. Mar 10, Available from:http://www.whqlibdoc.who.int/hq/2009/WHO_IER_PSP_2009.07_eng.pdf.
59. Wurtz R, Karajovic M, Dacumos E, Jovanovic B, Hanumadass M. Nosocomial infections in a burn intensive care unit. Burns. 1995;21:181-4.
60. Yokoe DS, Mermel LA, Deverick AJ, Kathleen AM, Burstin H, David CP, et al. Executive summary: a compendium of strategies to Prevent Healthcare-Associated Infections in Acute Care Hospitals. Infection Control and Hospital Epidemiology. 2008;29:S12-S21.

7

Section

Specialty Nursing

SECTION EDITOR: Yatin Mehta

18

CHAPTER

Cardiac Critical Care

Yatin Mehta, Bhanu P Zawar

ACUTE CORONARY SYNDROME

In coronary artery disease (CAD) atherosclerotic plaque builds up inside the coronary arteries and restricts the supply of blood (and therefore the delivery of oxygen) to the heart. Acute coronary syndrome (ACS) describes the range of various myocardial ischemic states that includes unstable angina, non-ST elevated myocardial infarction (NSTEMI), or ST-elevated myocardial infarction (STEMI). The diagnosis and classification of ACS is based on a thorough review of clinical features, including electrocardiogram (ECG) and biochemical markers of myocardial necrosis.

Principles of Management of Uncomplicated Acute Myocardial Infarction (AMI)

- Give oxygen to maintain $SpO_2 \geq 98\%$
- Good venous access
- Continuous monitoring of the patient
- Nitroglycerin or morphine to control pain. Nurses must assess for a drop in blood pressure or changes in pain score every five to ten minutes after administering nitroglycerin.
- Plan for early thrombolysis and give aspirin if not contraindicated [heparin if using recombinant tissue plasminogen activator (rTPA)]
- Early beta blockade
- Gradual mobilization of the patient.

Complication of AMI

- Cardiopulmonary arrest
- Continuing chest pain—may be ischemic or pericarditis in origin
- Heart failure
- Hypotension is usually from cardiogenic shock. Consider hypovolemia, e.g. post-diuretic or thrombolytic reaction
- Tachy/brady arrhythmias (heart block)
- Valve dysfunction predominantly acute mitral regurgitation (MR)
- Pericardial tamponade (rare)

- Ventricular septal defect (VSD) (unusual, often presents 2–5 days after infarct)
- Complication of thrombolytic therapy arrhythmias, anaphylactoid reaction.

Management of Complicated AMI

General

Give oxygen to maintain SpO_2 ≥98%. Appropriate and prompt monitoring indicated, e.g. ECG, SpO_2, blood pressure (BP), Swan Gang pulmonary artery (PAC), coronary angiography (CAG) and echocardiography. It is essential to evaluate patients with suspected ACS immediately to prevent potentially fatal clinical consequences. Early risk stratification can assist in planning whether a patient should be managed with either an early invasive strategy or an initial conservative strategy.

Early Thrombolysis

The rTPA followed by heparin should be given in preference to streptokinase. Arterial or central venous cannulation should not be delayed if clinically indicated. These procedures should be performed by an experienced operator to minimize the risk of bleeding before their administration. The subclavian route should be avoided due to risk of bleeding.

Cardiology consult should be sought promptly if a patient is admitted in pump failure, continuing pain or valve dysfunction. Insertion of intra-aortic balloon pump (IABP) should be considered as soon as possible in these conditions.

If patient is ischemic, nitrate and heparin infusion, aspirin, clopidogrel, calcium channel and beta blockers (unless contraindicated) should be administered. In patients presenting with STEMI, reperfusion therapy should be administered to all eligible patients with symptom onset within the prior 12 hours. So, CAG should be done at the earliest. If pericarditis is there consider nonsteroidal anti-inflammatory drugs (NSAIDs). Nurses need to assess for hypotension, decreased urine output, cough, hyperkalemia, and renal insufficiency in patients receiving angiotensinogen converting enzyme (ACE) inhibitors.

Management of Heart Failure

- Consider insertion of IABP.
- Tachyarrhythmias [e.g. Ventricular tachycardia (VT) or ventricular fibrillation (VF)]—antiarrhythmics, synchronized cardioversion.
- Bradycardia—atropine; consider transvenous or transcutaneous temporary pacing; more common in inferior wall AMI.
- Valve dysfunction—consider surgery.

- Pericardial tamponade—pericardial aspiration should be done.
- VSD—consider surgery/device closer in catheterization laboratory.

Drug Doses

- Morphine: 1–2 mg repeat SOS, consider antiemetic medication, e.g. ondansetron in addition.
- Streptokinase: 1.5 million units in 100 mL 0.9% saline slowly given over 1 hour.
- rTPA (Alteplase): 15 mg bolus, then 0.75 mg/kg (maximum 50 mg) over 30 minutes, then 0.5 mg/kg (maximum 35 mg) over 60 minutes.
- Reteplase: 10 units intravenous (IV) bolus + another 10 units 30 minutes later.
- Aspirin: 75–150 mg per oral (PO).
- Clopidogrel: 75 mg [consider 300 mg PO for ACS (acute coronary syndrome)].
- Atenolol: 50 mg PO once daily increasing to 100 mg if not hypotensive and heart rate (HR) exceeds 70 bpm or 5 mg slow IV bolus.
- Metoprolol: 25–50 mg PO BD (titrate to HR 60 bpm)
- NTG: 10–200 μg/min IV followed by infusion or 0.5–1 mg sublingual (SL).
- Diltiazem: 60 mg PO tid.
- Nifedipine: 5–10 mg SL/PO hourly.
- Atropine: 0.3 mg IV (maximum 2 mg).
- Lignocaine: 1 mg/kg slow IV bolus then 2–4 mg/min.
- Amiodarone: 150–300 mg in 10–20 mL in 5% dextrose then 1 mg/min × 6 hours, then 0.5 mg/min × 18 hours given preferably in central line as it produces thrombophlebitis.

Cardiac Markers

Troponin T and Troponin I: Cardiac troponins are biochemical markers of myocardial tissue damage. Troponin T and Troponin I are very specific and more sensitive than CPK-MB isozyme. These cardiac enzymes usually rises 4–8 hours after injury to the myocardium, and can provide prognostic information in a suspected case of ACS. Troponin T may be elevated with renal dysfunction, polydermatomyositis, etc.

CPK-MB Isoenzyme

This cardiac enzyme rises 4–6 hours after injury to the myocardium and peaks at 24 hours of injury. Elevation can be predictive of mortality. False positives result can occur with exercise, trauma, muscle disease, diabetes mellitus (DM), pulmonary thromboembolism (PE), myocarditis, end stage renal disease, and heart failure.

Invasive Strategy

Patient should be adequately prepared for CAG. Patient should be kept nil by mouth. Part preparation include preparation from umbilicus to knee, and from elbow to wrist. Peripheral venous cannulation should be done on left side as right radial artery may be used for CAG. Check consent for CAG and explain the procedure to patient or relatives also do not forget to ask for dye allergy. Send all routine investigations including viral markers (HbsAg, HCV). Patient should be catheterized and then shifted to catheterization laboratory as soon as possible.

Receiving Patient from Catheterization Laboratory

- Shift the patient to bed from stretcher.
- Check groins and sheaths.
- Check IV lines and start oxygen to maintain $SaO_2 \geq 98\%$.
- Connect sheaths to pressure monitors.
- Carry out orders and monitor vitals.
- Monitor ECG rhythm, BP, intake/output, ACT, oxygen saturation.
- Ensure about the CAG report and plan of care coronary artery bypass grafting (CABG), percutaneous transluminal coronary angioplasty (PTCA), discharge.
- Leg should be straight for 6 hours after sheath removal pressure dressing should be applied on sheath site and mobilize the patient only after that.
- Do not remove sheath if it is ordered by doctor, or there is hypotension (systolic BP <100 mm Hg), or there is hypertension (systolic BP >150 mm Hg), or there is brady/tachyarrhythmias, or activated clotting time (ACT) is >160 second.

Intra-aortic Balloon Pump

Intra-aortic balloon pump (IABP)(Fig. 1) is a mechanical circulatory assist device that is used to support the left heart pump function. IABP reduces cardiac work by decreasing afterload and increases coronary blood flow. Balloon is inflated during diastole (when the aortic valve is closed), thus increases aortic pressure during diastole and increases coronary arterial blood supply which is mainly during diastole. Balloon is deflated prior to and during early left ventricular ejection hence reducing aortic pressure and thus afterload of the heart. IABP may also have favorable effects on right-sided heart function by complex mechanisms including accentuation of right ventricle myocardial blood flow, unloading the left ventricle causing reduction in pulmonary hypertension and right ventricle afterload. IABP is placed in the descending thoracic aorta percutaneously from groin. It is connected to a central console that regulates the inflation or deflation of the IABP with the passage of helium gas. Helium is used as it is highly soluble in blood and prevents the

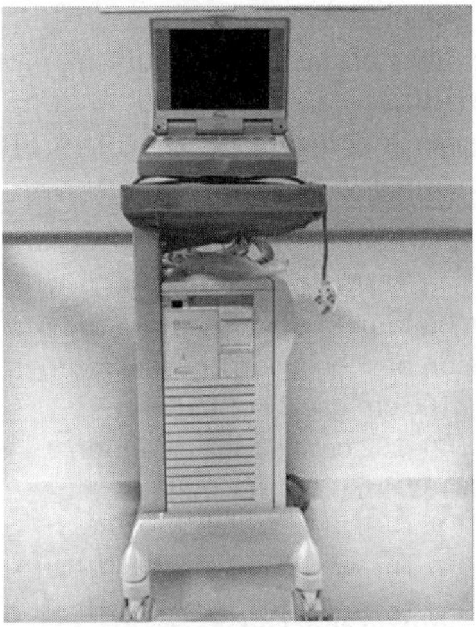

Fig. 1: Intra-aortic balloon pump

risk of air embolism if the catheter ruptures accidentally and has a low viscosity. Balloon catheter tip should be one centimeter lower to the origin of subclavian artery and lower end should be above the renal arteries.

The IABP has the following effects:

- Increases coronary arterial blood supply
- Increases myocardial oxygen supply
- Decreases myocardial work by reducing afterload
- Decreases myocardial total oxygen demand
- Increases systemic blood pressure
- Decreases pulmonary artery pressure.

Indicated in the following conditions if further medical treatment judged likely to be ineffective:

- Pump failure, imminent or frank. IABP is considered to be a class I indication American College of Cardiology/ American Heart Association (ACC/AHA) guidelines for the management of cardiogenic shock not rapidly reversed by pharmacological therapy
- Acute MR
- Unstable angina
- Stunned myocardium after myocardial infarction.

Also useful in:

- High-risk patients undergoing PTCA
- Ventricular arrhythmias refractory to conventional treatment
- Patients at high risk of cardiac decompensation during noncardiac surgery
- Bridge to cardiac transplantation.

Contraindications

- Severe aortic regurgitation (AR)
- Aortic dissection

- Prosthetic graft in the thoracic aorta
- Severe aortoiliac disease [e.g. aneurysm, peripheral vascular disease (PVD)]
- Practical aspects of use of IABP, i.e. lack of equipment or trained personnel.

IABP Size

The size of the balloon is dependent on the patients height to prevent occlusion of subclavian or renal arteries.

- For height <160 cm use 34 cc balloon
- For height 160–182 cm use 40 cc balloon
- For height >182 cm use 50 cc balloon.

Insertion

- Consent should be checked.
- Parts should be prepared from umbilicus to knees.
- Heparinize patient prior to insertion of catheter provided there are no contraindications.
- Fully collapse balloon by applying 30 mL vacuum with 60 mL syringe.
- Insert needle into femoral artery at an angle of 45° and pass it through both walls of artery. Withdraw needle until strong pulsatile jet of blood is obtained. IABP can also be inserted surgically using a transthoracic or translumbar approach, but this approach is associated with an increased periprocedural mortality.
- Pass guidewire through needle and advance until tip is in thoracic aorta. Wire should pass easily—Seldinger's technique.
- Pass sheath over wire in similar manner to insertion of PA catheter sheath.
- Pass balloon over guidewire through sheath (Seldinger's technique). Balloon must be inserted to at least the level of the manufacturer's mark (usually a double line).
- Balloon should be positioned so that the tip is about 1 cm distal to the origin of the left subclavian artery. If fluoroscopy is not available during insertion the distance from the angle of Louis down to the umbilicus and then to the femoral artery insertion site should be measured to approximate the distance the balloon should be advanced and the position should be checked on chest X-ray.
- Remove the wire and see for return of blood via central lumen that confirms that the tip is not subintimal and has not caused a dissection.
- Flush central lumen with heparin saline and connect to transducer to monitor intra-aortic pressure.
- Monitor Doppler ankle pressures and compare with preinsertion value.

Balloon Pump Timing

Using central aortic pressure waveform (from IABP tip) and ECG identify dicrotic notch (produced during aortic valve closure). Then determine the time delay between R wave and aortic valve opening and closure and enter these values into the pump. Turn on IABP and compare assisted and unassisted waveforms to determine whether timing is optimal or not. Inflation should be after the dicrotic notch and deflation should be before aortic valve opening. If inflation is too early or deflation too late the balloon waveform is superimposed to varying degrees over the LV systolic component (LV ejection) of the central aortic pressure waveform (i.e. inflation starts when the aortic valve is still open). This results in an increase in afterload to the left heart which result in premature valve closure and increase LV work and decreased cardiac output. In addition, it can increase intracardiac shunting in patients with a VSD. If inflation is too late or deflation is too early diastolic augmentation is suboptimal. Balloon inflation can be triggered by R wave, arterial waveform or pacing spike. Latter is a potentially lethal mode as loss of capture may result in balloon inflation during systole as the pump will continue to follow the pacing rate rather than the ventricular contraction rate.

Complications

During Insertion

- Failure to advance catheter beyond iliofemoral system because of atherosclerotic disease (most common complication)
- Aortic dissection and arterial perforation.

During Use

- Limb ischemia most common. Sufficiently severe to require removal of balloon in 11–27%.
- Sepsis. Relatively unusual but associated with high mortality. Positive blood cultures require prompt removal and culture of balloon tip and treatment with antibiotics.
- Thrombocytopenia can result from mechanical damage to the platelets, heparin administration, or both.
- Embolization of platelet aggregates from surface of balloon and cholesterol emboli.
- Balloon rupture leading to embolization of helium (2–4%). May be heralded by high balloon inflation pressures. Blood in connecting tubing is hallmark of rupture and requires immediate cessation of counterpulsation, placement of patient head down and IAB removal. Antibiotic cover should be broadened as the gas chamber of the balloon is not sterile.
- Small perforation in balloon membrane may allow small leak of blood into balloon lumen. Dry helium dessicates the

collected blood which then forms a hard pellet which may prevent removal of balloon except by surgical aortotomy.

During or Following Removal

- Hematoma
- False aneurysm
- Arteriovenous (AV) fistula.

Nursing Care of the Patient Undergoing IABP Therapy

1. Only nurses who have been trained in the timing and trouble shooting of the IABP should be caring for these patients. The nurse/patient ratio for a patient with an IABP is 1:1.
   Rationale: This is to provide safe, consistent levels of nursing care for IABP patients. The nurse assigned to relieve for breaks will be approved to care for the patient on the IABP.
2. Ensure that a set of skin and external leads are connected and functional. Select the desired ECG source from waveform selector in the IABP controls.
   Rationale: A back-up triggering mode must be readily available. Adjust trigger modes as required to ensure balloon pumping.
3. The ECG trigger will be used for most situations. Pressure trigger is a suitable trigger if the ECG is temporarily lost, there is arrhythmia or if the patient has no ECG rhythm and is receiving cardiopulmonary resuscitation (CPR). The pacemaker trigger should be avoided as explained above. After changing the trigger mode the assist button must be pressed to resume pumping.
   Rationale: Trigger modes may require changing to ensure optimal balloon function. Adjust by using the arrows in the auxiliary trigger option. ECG trigger mode will work well for patients being paced. The pacemaker trigger modes will only work for fixed rate pacing. If the patient is in a pacemaker trigger mode, the pump will ignore native beats and only operate with paced impulses.
4. A previously prepared and zeroed transducer is connected to the aortic arterial line of the balloon and then to the IABP. This should be secured level with the patient's mid-axillary line. This position should be rechecked hourly and with each patient repositioning.
   Rationale: The pressure module provides an alternate blood pressure source in the event that the bedside monitor should fail. The IABP pressure should be the one that is treated.
5. The pressures are to be recorded on the ICU flowchart every hour. These include assisted peak systolic pressure (APSP), balloon aortic end diastolic pressure (BAEDP), diastolic

augmentation (DA), and unassisted aortic end diastolic pressure (EDP). The pressures from the IABP are the ones that should be treated. Vasoactive drugs should be titrated according to the mean blood pressure (MAP) from the IABP console. The BP from the IABP console should be used when calculating hemodynamics.

Rationale: When the IABP is timed adequately the diastolic blood pressure (DBP) is augmented to be higher than the systolic blood pressure (SBP). The SBP will be the highest pressured on the bedside monitor. If the balloon is successful at augmenting the DBP above the SBP, the SBP displayed by the bedside monitor will actually be the augmented DBP.

The IABP console differentiates between the SBP, augmented pressure and end diastolic pressure. It will also display assisted and unassisted systole and diastole if the pump is placed in 1:2 or 1:3 mode.

6. Assess capillary refill and pedal pulses hourly. Assess capillary refill and left radial pulse at the start of each shift and hourly. Notify the physician of any change from the previous hour. Document on flow sheet and nursing note.

   Rationale: The balloon catheter or thrombus can obstruct flow to the distal extremities. If the balloon migrates too high, it can obstruct flow to the left subclavian artery.

The following must be done each hour by assigned nurse:

- Every hour, fast flush on standby to keep clots from forming at the tip of the IABP catheter. This may not be required if their is a continuous flush device (check the pressure in the bag).
- Record IABP pressures hourly, these include APSP, BAEDP, DA, EDP.
- Use minimal tubing necessary in the transducer to insure accuracy.
- Listen between second and third intercostal space for placement, the sound should be in the same location. At times, the IABP can migrate from its intended location.
- Check urine output. The balloon can occlude the renal artery leading to reduced urine output.
- Check the left radial artery pulsation.
- Keep limb warm and check for signs of ischemia.
- Keep ACT between 180–200 seconds.
- Limb ischemia is very common. Check dorsalis pedis pulse manually or by using Doppler hourly and record. Call the doctor stat if in doubt.

Before Removal of IABP

- Stop heparin two hours before.
- Check ACT. If still prolonged, consider reversal of heparin with protamine.

- Put IABP on weaning mode, i.e. 1:1 → 1:2 →1:3.
- Make sure that patient is hemodynamically stable.

After Removal of IABP

- Keep blood pressure low.
- If bleeding, press one inch above the site. Do not press on site.

FURTHER READING

1. Bojar RM. Manual of Perioperative Care in Adult Cardiac Surgery. 2011 Wiley-Blackwell. 978-1-4443-3143-1.
2. Bradley D, Creswell LL, Hogue Jr CW, Epstein AE, Prystowsky EN, Daoud EG. American College of Chest Physicians Guidelines for the Prevention and Management of Postoperative Atrial Fibrillation After Cardiac Surgery. Chest. 2005;128, Suppl: 39S-47S.
3. Crossley AW. Peri-operative Shivering. Anaesthesia. 1992;47:193-5.
4. Daoud EG, Strictberger A, Mab C, et al. Preoperative amiodarone as prophylaxis against atrial fibrillation after heart surgery. N Engl J Med. 1997;337:1785-91.
5. Frank SM, Fleisher LA, Breslow MJ, Higgins MS, Olson KF, Kelly S, et al. Perioperative Maintenance of Normothermia Reduces the Incidence of Morbid Cardiac Events. A Randomized Clinical Trial. JAMA. 1997;277:1127-34.
6. Ho KM, Tan JA. Benefit is and Risks of Maintaining Normothermia During Cardiopulmonary Bypass in Adlut Cardiac Surgery: A Systemic Review. Cardiovasc Ther. 2009;29:260-79.
7. Koniari I, Apostolakis E, Rogkakou C, Baikoussis NG, Dougenis D. Pharmacologic Prophylaxis for Arial Fibrillation Following Cardiac Surgery: A Systemic Review. J Cardiothorac Surg. 2010;5:121.
8. Korff S, Katus HA, Giannitsis E. Differential diagnosis of elevated troponins. Heart. 2006;92:987-93.
9. McKhann GM, Grega MA, Borowicz LM, Baumgartner WA, Selnes OA. Stroke and Encephalopathy After Cardiac Surgery. An Update. Stroke. 2006;37:562-71.
10. Mehta Y, Kumar S. New horizon in cardiac surgery (Editorial). Ind J Crit Care Med. 2004;8:11-3.
11. Mehta Y, Singh R. Cognitive Dysfunction After Cardiac Surgery. Review. J Alzheim Dis. 2010;22:S115-S20.
12. Miller RD. Miller's anaesthesia. In: Nyhan D, Johns RA (Eds). Anesthesia for Cardiac Surgery. Elsevier. 1991/2007.
13. Mitchell LB. The CCS Atrial Fibrillation Guidelines Committee. Canadian Cardiovascular Society Atrial Fibrillation Guidelines 2010: Prevention and Treatment of Atrial Fibrillation Following Cardiac Surgery. Can J Cardiol. 2011;27:91-7.
14. O'Gara PT, Kushner FG, Ascheim DD, et al. ACCF/AHA guideline for the management of Stelevation myocardial infarction: A report of the American College of Cardiology Foundation/American Heart Association Task Force on Practice Guidelines. J Am Coll Cardiol. 2013;61:e78-e140.
15. Pradeep A, Rajagopalam S, Kolli HK, Patel N, Venuto R, Lohr J, et al. High Volumes of Intravenous Fluid During Cardiac surgery are Associated with Increased Mortality. HSR Proceedings in Intensive Care and Cardiovascular Anesthesia. 2010:2:287-96.

16. Rajagopalan S, Mascha E, Na J, Sessler DI. The Effectis of Mild Perioperative Hypothermia on Blood Loss and Transfusion Requirement. Anesthesiology. 2008;108:71-7.
17. Reichlin T, Hochholzer W, Bassetti S, et al. Early diagnosis of myocardial infarction with sensitive cardiac troponin assays. N Engl J Med. 2009;361:858-67.
18. Ryan TJ, Antman EM, Brooks NH, et al. 1999 update: ACC/AHA Guidelines for the Management of Patients with Acute Myocardial-Infarction: Executive Summary and Recommendations: A Report of the American College of Cardiology/American Heart Association Task Force on Practice Guidelines (Committee on Management of Acute Myocardial Infarction). Circulation. 1999;100:1016-30.
19. Sessler DI. Complications and Treatment of Mild Hypothermia. Anesthesiology. 2001;95:531-43.
20. Springhouse Nurse's Drug Guide 2007, 8th edn. Philadelphia: Lippincott Williams and Wilkins; 2006.
21. Thygesen K, Alpert JS, Jaffe AS, et al. Third universal definition of myocardial infarction. Circulation. 2012;126:2020-35.
22. Thygesen K, Alpert JS, Jaffe AS, et al. Third universal definition of myocardial infarction. Circulation. 2012;126:2020-35.
23. Walls JT, Boley TM, Curtis JJ, Silver D. Heparin induced thrombocytopenia in patients undergoing intra-aortic balloon pumping after open heart surgery. ASAIO J. 1992;38:M574-6.
24. Zimmerman N, Gams E, Hohlfeld T. Aspirin in Coronary Artery Bypass Surgery: New Aspects of and Alternatives for an Old Antithrombotic Agent. Review. Eur J Cardiothorac Surg. 2008;34:93-108.

19

CHAPTER

Postoperative Care of Coronary Artery Bypass Graft Patients

Manish Munjal, Navneet Mehta

INTRODUCTION

The purpose of this chapter is to discuss hand-off of care from operating room (OR) team to intensive care unit (ICU) team and approach to common problems that occur in ICU.

Traditional cardiac surgery is performed via a median sternotomy incision on a quiet bloodless heart with the use of a cardiopulmonary bypass (CPB) or heart lung machine, which maintains total body oxygenation and perfusion despite cardiac arrest. After CPB is initiated, injection of hyperkalemic cardioplegia solution directly into the coronary circulation stops the heart. Cardioplegia also provides necessary nutrients for myocardial preservation despite the absence of cardiac blood flow. Traditional surgical approaches are associated with varying degrees of hypothermia, coagulopathy, hemodilution (resulting in edema and tissue edema), and postoperative mechanical ventilation.

Some patients of coronary artery disease can be operated for CABG without going on the CPB pump. Such surgeries are called off pump or beating heart surgeries. Minimally invasive cardiac surgery (MICS) modifies or more of the foregoing techniques to accomplish similar surgical options through small surgical incisions with or without CPB (i.e. off pump). These changes have been shown to reduce blood requirements, length of ICU/hospital stay and resource use. Additionally endoscopic and robotic surgery are likely to become common in the days to come.

Checklist before Receiving Patient from Operation Theater

- Keep sterile bed with all equipment ready.
- Monitor ready with modules—electrocardiography (ECG), intra-aortic balloon pump (IABP), central venous pressure (CVP), SPO_2, temperature.
- Ventilator ready checked and calibrated.
- Emergency drugs and the emergency cart be prepared.
- Pacemaker standby.

- External defibrillator charged and checked.
- Availability of special bed for patient at high-risk of developing pressure ulcer.

Handover of Care from Operating Room Team to Intensive Care Unit Team

Best hand-offs occur when they are structured, standardized and use check list.

- Details of the patient—name, sex, salient feature of history.
- All preoperative investigations including angiogram be submitted.
- Preoperative medications.
- Operation performed and problems encountered.
- Ejection fraction of patient, blood group, and allergy.
- Number of pacing wires and chest drains.
- Current drugs infusions and plans for tapering.
- Pacemaker and anti-arrhythmic information.
- Fluids and blood administered, urine output, OT fluid balance.
- Sedatives administered and plans for awakening and weaning.
- Antibiotics administered and timing.
- Last arterial blood gas, hematocrit.
- Availability of blood products.
- Any metabolic abnormalities (glucose, acid-base and electrolyte).

Staff should take over of the patient in an organized way. The following should be checked.

Breathing

Patient is connected to the ventilator.

- Look for chest movement.
- Auscultate and confirm air entry to both the lungs.
- Ask the accompanying anesthetist about the ventilator setting and set them accordingly. The usual setting are:
  - Breath rate of 10–12 breaths/min.
  - Initial FIO_2 of 1.0 (100% O_2).
  - Tidal volume: 8–10 mL/kg.
- PEEP as per protocol.
- Depending on ABG report, settings are changed. Aim to maintain PaO_2 of 90–120 mm Hg and $PaCO_2$ of 35–40 mm Hg.
- Sedation to be started as per protocol.
- Endotracheal and oral suction should be performed before chest X-ray.

Circulation

- Attach radial/femoral artery line to the transducer and ensure satisfactory pressure.

- Attach PA or CVP pressure line (if present) to transducer, exclude air before flushing.
- Always perform the zeroing of the pressure transducer.

The things to check are:

- Attach ECG and check for rate, rhythm, and ST-segment changes.
- Blood gases are done every 2–4 hours and electrolytes, lactate, glucose and hemoglobin are checked.
- Pulmonary artery pressure/central venous pressure—measure the pulmonary capillary wedge pressure (PCWP), cardiac output (CO), systemic vascular resistance (SVR). Cardiac output and parameters checked every 2 hours for first 6 hours then every 4 hours.
- Temperature probe—if temperature less than 37°C warming blanket of radiant heat should be placed.

Maintaining Normothermia

Patients usually arrive in the ICU with lower body temperatures. This fall in temperature during cardiac surgery or from end of CPB until arrival in the ICU is due to the cool temperatures in the operation room, poor peripheral perfusion and anesthesia-induced inhibition of normal thermoregulation. Hypothermia also increases the SVR which increases myocardial afterload and myocardial oxygen demand. Drugs that cause vasodilation may improve peripheral perfusion, decrease in SVR and decrease in myocardial oxygen demand. Hypothermia also precipitates shivering, thereby increasing CO_2 production and oxygen consumption, and predisposes to ventricular arrhythmias (ventricular fibrillation) and coagulation cascade impairment. Therefore, rewarming should be hastened by forced-air warming blankets, heated humidifiers in the ventilator circuit and warmed infusion of fluids. The use of other types of warming blankets or radiant heading hoods can also be considered.

Drugs

Most of the patient who have undergone heart surgery are shifted from the OT on some IV drugs (inotropes, vasodilators).

- Hourly charting of inotropes to be done and orders asked about tapering.

Fluids

Patients are kept nil by mouth till 2–4 hours after extubation. IV maintenance fluids are started at the rate of 1–1.5 mL/kg/h:

- Maintain potassium at 4.0–4.5 mmoL/L.
- Colloid to maintain PCWP at 8–15 mm Hg.
- Blood to keep hematocrit at >27–30%.
- Magnesium supplementation to avoid hypomagnesemia.

- Maintain urine output at >1.0 mL/kg/hour.
- Analgesia as per unit protocol.

(In diabetic patient, dextrose infusions should be neutralized with insulin).

Investigations

A set of investigations is done within 30 minutes of arrival in ICU.

- Arterial blood gas
- Chest X-ray

Chest drain tubes are left in the chest before closure. Unclamp the chest tube and these are connected to underwater seals to prevent pneumothorax.

If excessive bleeding, patient is taken back to operation theater to control the bleeding.

In adult patient inform surgeon/anesthetist if bleeding is significant when:

- More than 400 mL/h for 1 hour
- More than 300 mL/h for 2–3 hours
- More than 200 mL/h for 4 hours.

(CPB may induce coagulation abnormalities in the patient. These may be the cause of excessive bleeding).

Anticoagulation Protocols

Valve Surgery

Patient undergone mechanical valve replacement are put on oral anticoagulant (Warfarin or Acitrom) as soon as oral feeds are started (48–72 hours).

- Initial anticoagulation is maintained with heparin.
- Heparin is stopped once the desired INR is achieved.

Coronary artery bypass graft: Aspirin in low doses are started as soon as oral feeds are started. Clopidogrel may be started in endarterectomy cases.

General Care of Patient

- Position—head end elevated at 30 degree
- Prevention of infection
  - Wash hands
  - Wear sterile gloves for all procedures
- Infected waste are disposed according to guidelines
- Neurological assessment—to check whether patient is obeying command or not, whether the patient is moving all four limbs.

Common Complications after Cardiac Surgery

1. Atrial arrhythmias are the most common complication after cardiac surgery, occurring in 25% to 60% of patients. Advanced age is the most important risk factor for atrial fibrillation, as well as prior atrial fibrillation and combined bypass graft/valve surgery. Evidence indicates that prophylactic beta-blocker or amiodarone therapy is effective. Maintain the electrolytes in normal range.

2. Respiratory failure: It is most common postoperative complication. Postoperative pain exacerbates this. Respiratory failure can present as hypoxemia, hypercarbia, or both. Atelectasis is a universal finding owing to lung under inflation during CPB and may contribute to pneumonia if pulmonary hygiene efforts are inadequate. Patients may require BIPAP or CPAP therapy and aggressive physiotherapy.
3. Cardiac tamponade: Excessive mediastinal bleeding with inadequate drainage or sudden massive bleeding can result in tamponade.
4. Pneumothorax.
5. Pleural effusions are also common because of extensive dissection required in harvesting the left or right internal mammary artery as a bypass conduit.
6. Fluid overload is related to large—volume infusions and the antidiuretic hormonal response to surgery, and it requires aggressive diuresis to achieve baseline weight.
7. Significant neurological deficit occur in 2–3% of patients undergoing coronary artery bypass surgery, including strokes, transient ischemic attack, and coma.
   Perioperative strokes can be attributed to microemboli of air or fat, mural thrombus, or disruption of atheromatous plaque by the aortic cross clamp. A reduced incidence of neurological impairment has been noticed after MICS, attributed in part to avoidance of aortic cross clamping. Although many patients exhibit substantial recovery from stoke, postoperative mortality rate and length of stay are increased.
8. Sternal wound infection occurs in fewer than 2% of patients. Risk factors include obesity, immune-suppression, bilateral internal mammary artery and uncontrolled diabetes. Strict control of perioperative blood glucose levels using continuous intravenous. Insulin has been shown to reduce infection rates and mortality significantly in diabetic patients.

20
CHAPTER

Neurocritical Care

Kapil Zirpe, Sushma Gurav

NEUROLOGICAL EMERGENCIES

Neurocritical care focuses on the care of critically ill patients with primary or secondary neurosurgical and neurological problems and was initially developed to manage postoperative neurosurgical patients. It expanded thereafter to the management of patients with traumatic brain injury (TBI), intracranial hemorrhage and complications of subarachnoid hemorrhage; including vasospasm, elevated intracranial pressure (ICP), etc.

In the neurocritical care unit, nurse is a important member of highly collaborative and multidisciplinary team. This multidisciplinary team supports the patient and family to achieve realistic goals.

Early identification of patients at risk of life-threatening neurological illness and to prevent further deterioration is the role of nurse in the neurocritical unit. Her role is to be supportive to the patient, providing brief explanation, emotional and psychological support as necessary.

ASSESSMENT OF UNCONSCIOUS PATIENT

In the initial assessment of coma, it is common to judge by spontaneous actions, response to vocal stimuli and response to painful stimuli; this is known as the AVPU (alert, vocal stimuli, painful stimuli, unconscious) scale. The most common scales used for rapid assessment are:

- The Glasgow Coma Scale (GCS), which aims to record the conscious state of a person, in initial as well as continuing assessment. When a patient is assessed and the resulting score is either 14 (original scale) or 15 (the more widely used modified or revised scale), this means 'normal'; while if a patient is unable to voluntarily open their eyes, does not have a sleep-wake cycle, is unresponsive in spite of strong sensory (painful) or verbal stimuli and who generally scores between 3 and 8 on the Glasgow Coma Scale, (s)he is considered to be in coma (Table 1).

Table 1: Glasgow Coma Score

Score	*Eye opening*	*Best verbal response*	*Best verbal response*
6	—	—	Obeys command
5	—	Oriented	Localizes pain
4	Spontaneously	Confused	Purposeful movement/ flexion withdrawal
3	To speech	Inappropriate words	Decerebrate flexion
2	To pain	Incomprehensible	Decerebrate extension
1	Does not open	Silent	No response

Maximum score is 15 ($E_4V_5M_6$)

- Pupillary functions may be normal if the lesion is above or rostral to the midbrain, while if the injury is diffuse, e.g. global ischemia, the pupillary abnormality is bilateral.
- Recording the pupil size is important for a variety of reasons fixed or irregular pupils imply a focal midbrain lesion pinpoint reactive pupils occur in global hypoxic ischemic insult with pontine damage, or poisoning with opiates and cholinergic active materials bilateral fixed and dilated pupils can reflect central herniation or global hypoxic ischemic or poisoning with barbiturates, scopolamine, and atropine.
- Unilateral dilated pupil suggests compression of the third cranial nerve and midbrain, which necessitates an immediate search for a potentially correctable abnormality to avoid irreversible injury.
- In case of post-cardiac arrest coma, if pupils remain non-reactive for more than 6–8 hours after resuscitation, the prognosis for neurological recovery is generally guarded

Components of Neurological Examination

- Level of consciousness
- Mental status
- Cranial nerve examination
- Motor system
- Sensory system
- Cerebellar
- Pupil size and reaction.

Component of Care

- Maintain airway
- Observe vital signs
- Maintain personal hygeine
- Provide sufficient nutrition by giving tube feeding/ intravenous (IV) fluids.
- Maintain urinary and bowel movement
- Prevention of contracture.

Specific nursing care to be carried out according to the diagnosis, drugs used and surgery if done. Nursing care should also aim at the early rehabilitation of the patient with minimal complications.

CONCEPT OF RISING INTRACRANIAL PRESSURE

Presentation

Headache, seizure, increasing drowsiness, vomiting, dizziness, visual disturbance, seizures.

Signs

Listlessness, irritability, drowsiness, falling pulse (bradycardia), rising BP, coma, irregular breathing (Cheyne-Stokes breathing), change in pupils size, decorticate progressing to decerebrate posturing, change in GCS score , craniotomy defect tensed.

Causes

Space occupying lesion (SOL):	Primary/metastatic tumors
Increased capillary permeability:	Head injury meningoencephalitis, encephalopathy, brain abscess
Hemorrhage:	EDH, SDH, SAH, intracerebral, IVH
Cell death:	Post arrest hypoxia
Obstruction:	Hydrocephalus

Treatment

Goal: Decrease ICP and avert secondary injury.

Asset-based Community Development (ABCD) Approach

Urgent neurosurgical intervention for definitive treatment of increase ICP.

Other Measures

- Elevate the head of bed to 30–45 degrees
- Ventilate if GCS ≤8, airway unprotected or excessively agitated
- Hyperventilation (bridge therapy before taking for surgery, benefit for only 4–6 hours)
- Osmotic agents, e.g. Mannitol—20% solution 1–2 g/kg over 10–20 minutes
- Steroids not effective except in edema surrounded tumors and encephalitis
- Jugular bulb venous saturation (SjO_2) and lactate may be useful.

CARE IN SPECIFIC EMERGENCIES

Traumatic Brain Injury

Goal of Management

Preventing secondary injury due to hypotension episode, hypoxia and preserving cerebral functioning and assisting individuals to return to society at maximum level of independences.

- Frequent assessment of neurological signs
- Early recognition of complications
- Control of cerebral edema and increase ICP.

Outcome after traumatic brain injury depends upon the initial severity of the injury, age, the extent of any subsequent complications, and how these are managed. Much of the early management of traumatic brain injury falls upon emergency room staff, primary care and ambulance services prior to hospital admission. Most patients who attend hospital after a traumatic brain injury do not develop life-threatening complications in the acute stage. However, in a small but important subgroup, the outcome is made worse by failure to detect promptly and deal adequately with complications.

General Rules

- A traumatic brain injury should be discussed with neurosurgery when:
  - A CT scan in a general hospital shows a recent intracranial lesion.
  - A patient fulfils the criteria for CT scanning but this cannot be done within an appropriate period.
  - Whatever the result of the CT scan, the patient has clinical features that suggest that specialist neurological assessment, monitoring, or management are appropriate. Reasons include:
    - Persistent coma (GCS <9, no eye opening) after initial resuscitation
    - Confusion persisting for more than 4 hours
    - Deterioration in level of consciousness after admission (a sustained decrease of one point in the motor or verbal GCS subscores, or 2 points on the eye opening subscale of the GCS)
    - Persistent focal neurological signs
    - A seizure without full recovery
    - Compound depressed fracture
    - Suspected or definite penetrating injury
    - A CSF leak or other sign of base of skull fracture.
- Keep sodium >140 mmol/L. A fall in serum sodium produces an osmotic gradient across the blood-brain barrier, and aggravates cerebral edema.
- Avoid hyperglycemia (treat blood glucose >11 mmol/L). Hyperglycemia increases cerebral lactic acidosis, which may aggravate ischemic brain injury.

- Feed via an orogastric tube. Gastric motility agents can be given as required.
- Use TED stockings; avoid low-dose heparin.
- Apply 15–30° head-up tilt with head kept in neutral position; this may improve CPP.
- No parenteral hypotonic fluid must be given.

Patient who require surgery will be managed with same nursing protocol as for a craniotomy.

If basal skull fracture suspected avoid suction through nasal passage and avoid nasal insertion of feeding or endotracheal tube and look for facial palsy, deafness, nasal rhinorrhea, otorrhea, ecchymosis of temporal bone.

Primary Brain Injuries

Ischemic brain injury: either global, which includes cardiac arrest or anoxia, or regional ischemic brain injury, which includes vasospasm, compression of blood vessels or stroke.

Stroke can be classified into ischemic and hemorrhagic strokes. Ischemic stroke accounts for 80% of all strokes and can be further classified into thrombotic or embolic stroke; ischemic thrombotic stroke accounts for 77% while ischemic embolic stroke constitutes the remainder.

Hemorrhagic strokes constitute 10–20% of all strokes, and can be further classified into two types, the intracerebral hemorrhage that constitutes up to 75% and the subarachnoid hemorrhage that makes up the other 25%.

Acute ischemic stroke is the third leading cause of permanent disability in adults worldwide, so understanding the pathogenesis of ischemic stroke is mandatory. Despite great strides in understanding the pathophysiology of cerebral ischemia, therapeutic options remain limited. Only recombinant tissue plasminogen activator (rTPA) for thrombolysis is currently approved for use in the management of acute ischemic stroke. However, its use is limited by its short therapeutic window (3–4.5 hours), complications from the risk of hemorrhage, and the potential damage from reperfusion injury.

Central nervous system (CNS) infections: Acute onset fever with altered mental status is a problem commonly encountered by the physician in the emergency setting. CNS infections are the most common cause of nontraumatic disturbed consciousness. The etiologic agents may be viruses, bacteria, or parasites. Central nervous system infections are classified into categories beginning with those in immunocompetent hosts followed by infection with the human immunodeficiency virus (HIV) and its opportunistic infections.

The viruses responsible for most cases of acute encephalitis in immunocompetent hosts are herpes viruses, arboviruses, and enteroviruses. Neurotropic herpes viruses that cause encephalitis predominantly in immunocompetent hosts include herpes simplex virus 1 (HSV-1) and 2 (HSV-2), and Epstein-

Barr virus (EBV). Cytomegalovirus (CMV) and varicella-zoster virus (VZV) may in some situations cause encephalitis in immunocompetent patients, but more commonly they produce an opportunistic infection in immunocompromised individuals, such as those with HIV infection, organ transplant recipients, or other patients using immunosuppressive drugs.

In a good number of cases, infection is iatrogenic, being introduced in the course of cerebral or spinal surgery, during the placement of a ventriculoperitoneal shunt or rarely through a lumbar puncture needle. Nowadays, nosocomial infections are as frequent as the non-hospital-acquired variety.

Compressive Brain Injury

For example, tumors and cerebral brain edema are considered as important causes for impairment of the level of consciousness. During tumor growth, cerebral tissues adjacent to the tumor and nearby venules are compressed, which results in elevation of capillary pressure, particularly in the cerebral white matter, and there is a change in cerebral blood flow and consequently intracranial pressure. At that stage, the tumor begins to displace tissue, which eventually leads to displacement of tissue at a distance from the tumor, resulting in false localizing signs.

Secondary Brain Injuries

Secondary brain injuries include renal coma, hepatic coma, salt and water imbalance, disturbance of glucose metabolism, other endocrinal causes of coma, disturbances of calcium and magnesium metabolism, drug intoxication and other material intoxication, not only drug toxicity, hypertensive and metabolic encephalopathies, sleep apnea syndromes and other ventilator disturbances. Mechanisms of secondary brain injury include hypoxia, hypoperfusion, reperfusion injury with free radical formations, release of excitatory amino acids and harmful mediators from injured cells, electrolyte and acid-based changes from systemic or regional ischemia. The primary goal in managing neurologically compromised patients includes stabilizing the brain through the maintenance of oxygen delivery via the following parameters:

- Assuring systemic oxygen transport and adequate oxygenation, maintaining hemoglobin level (at approximately 10 g/dL or more) and cardiac output.
- Assuring optimal mean arterial pressure (MAP). Many insults are associated with hypertension, which may be a physiologic compensation, so excessive lowering of blood pressure may induce secondary ischemia. In general, systolic pressure should be treated when more than 200 mm Hg or MAP when more than 125 mm Hg. Cautious reduction in mean arterial pressure by only 25% is recommended.
- Avoiding prophylactic or routine hyperventilation—a decrease in extracellular brain pH may produce vasocon-

striction in responsive vessels and reduce CBF to already ischemic zones. This applies to patients with head trauma in whom routine hyperventilation is no longer considered desirable; brief hyperventilation may be lifesaving in the patient with herniation, pending the institution of other methods to lower elevated ICP.

- Assuring euvolemia. Hypervolemia may also be helpful when vasoconstriction is suspected, as in the setting of subarachnoid hemorrhage.
- Consideration should be given to administering intravenous lidocaine 1.5 mg/kg or intravenous thiopental (5 mg/kg) to blunt the rise in ICP associated with intubation.
- Nimodipine should be instituted immediately in patients with SAH and is advocated by some in patients with subarachnoid bleeding after head trauma. Nimodipine probably improves outcome by decreasing calcium mediated neuronal toxicity.
- Using normal saline as the primary maintenance fluid; dextrose administration is usually avoided unless the patient is hypoglycemic; hypotonic solutions should also be avoided.
- Assessing and treating coagulation defects.
- Sedation and/or neuromuscular blockade after intubation may be required to control harmful agitation.
- If seizure occurs, it should be aggressively treated.
- Titration of the ICP and cerebral perfusion pressure.

INTRACRANIAL HEMORRHAGE—EDH/SDH/SAH/ICH

Nursing Management

- Patient to be kept in complete bed rest
- Head end elevated to 30–45 degrees
- Patient to be turned every 2 hourly
- Neurological sign to be recorded hourly (GCS, papillary size and reaction to light, developing neurological deficits or focal signs)
- Vital signs to be recorded frequently
- Analgesic to prevent/treat headache
- Observe for seizure activity
- Implement early nutrition
- Emotional support, provides communication
- Education, provides knowledge of patients condition and treatment to the next of kin.

CEREBROVASCULAR ACCIDENTS/STROKE

Nursing Management

- Care during acute phase
- Maintenance of body functions and prevention of complications

- Psychological needs
- Rehabilitation
- Discharge planning and continuity of care.

Care During Acute Phase

ABCD approach

- Thrombolysis if acute ischemic stroke if patient arrives in emergency during the window period (<4.5 hours after symptoms started), monitor blood pressure.
- Maintain clear airway for adequate ventilators and to prevent hypoxia
- Observe and record her vital signs and neurological status as frequently as necessary
- Observe and recorded the rate, rhythm, depth of respirations
- Temperature—hyperthermia damage to hypothalamus
- Level of consciousness—GCS
- Pupillary reaction
- Draw the blood for necessary investigation
- Care of patient while on heparin
- Monitor coagulation studies and maintain therapeutic range using INR parameter
- If patient in altered sensorium—maintain nothing by mouth status, Enteral feed to the given to compensate nutritional needs after stabilization.

Postacute Phase

After return to consciousness, coughing and swallowing reflexes may be impaired.

Maintain Safe Environment

- Padded cot site
- Change position frequently.

Establish effective communication

The patient attempt to communicate should be supported.

Physiotherapy

Encourage mobilization/prevent contractures.

Elimination

- Patient may be unable to control bladder and bowel function
- Observe for incontinence of urine and feces
- Institute bladder and bowel training if necessary.

Psychological Needs

- Reassure patient and family
- Neglect burst of emotions
- Anticipate his need and meet them in time.

Rehabilitation

- Start as soon as patient is stabilized
- Encourage patient to do as much of his/her personal hygiene as possible

- Teach activity of daily living—dressing, toileting, bathing, eating, gait training
- Encourage family participation.

Spinal Injury

Spinal cord injury is usually associated with vertebral column injury.

The primary survey for injured patients consists of the ABCDs:

A—airway with cervical spine control

B—breathing with particular attention to cervical area and intercostal muscles

C—circulation, establishing intravenous access, checking pulses, stopping external bleeding

D—disability; a quick neurologic exam for responsiveness and pupils size and reaction.

While transferring the patient use firm structure of any improvised method to prevent the further injury to vertebral column and spinal cord. (Maintain alignment and immobilization with long spine board). Begin skin care of pressure areas as early as possible.

In Hospital Care

Frequent examination

To assess—Spinal cord dysfunction/Regaining of lost function.

Cardiovascular status

Heart rate, rhythm, BP (Autonomic dysfunction).

Assess respiratory status

- Early identification of respiratory dysfunction
- Provide nutrition and DVT prophylaxis.

Pressure sore

- Frequent turning and skin assessment
- Monitor bowel movement
- Emotional support and provide knowledge of patient condition and treatment.

Seizures

Goal

To coordinate multidisciplinary approach aimed to provide safety and prevent injury to patient which includes.

Airway Protection

Keep the patient in lateral position to prevent aspiration

Protection from body injury by

- Bed lowest possible
- Providing side rails.

Documenting vitals signs, time of onset and completion of seizures and body parts involved in the pattern of involvement and progressing.

Causes

Hypoxemia, hypoglycemia, hypocalcemia, space occupying lesion (SOL), metabolic and toxic disorders, drug withdrawal, (alcohol, anticonvulsants), trauma, infection meningoencephilitis.

Following Seizures

Patient in postictal phase are often confused, disoriented and at times unconscious, so they require continuous neurological, hemodynamic assessment.

Specific Treatment

ABCD approach

- Blood glucose measured, anticonvulsant level
- Cerebral edema managed with sedation, hyperventilation, osmotic diuretics
- In patient with SOL high dose dexamethasone
- Thiamine 100 mg IV to alcoholics
- Surgery for space occupying lesion, e.g. blood clot, tumor

Status epilepticus

Status epilepticus is defined as more than 30 minutes of continuous seizure activity or recurrent seizure activity without an intervening period of consciousness. It is an emergency and must be treated immediately with anticonvulsants such as Lorazepam (0.1 mg/kg IV at 2 mg/min maximum 4 mg) or phenytoin 20 mg/kg at 50 mg/min. Initial priority airway protection, if necessary intubate.

21

CHAPTER

Liver Failure

Deepak Govil

CARE OF PATIENTS WITH LIVER DYSFUNCTION AND FAILURE

Liver is one organ that subserves several functions. It controls several metabolic pathways and participates in digestion of ingested food. It is also involved in immunological protection and detoxifying drugs and toxins. Liver failure is the inability of the liver to perform its normal synthetic and metabolic function as part of normal physiology.

Anatomy and Physiology

Liver is the largest internal organ weighing approximately 1200–1600 g in the adults. It receives 25% of the cardiac output through a dual blood supply of hepatic artery and portal vein. 75% of the hepatic blood flow is contributed to by the portal vein. Anatomically it has four lobes. The right and left are the major lobes and the quadrate and caudate lobes are the minor lobes. Functionally, the liver has 8 segments with their own blood supply and venous/bile drainage. The bile produced by liver helps in absorption of fats from the intestine.

Liver Dysfunction/Failure

Liver dysfunction can be acute or chronic. Chronic liver failure usually occurs in the context of cirrhosis, which may have several possible causes, such as excessive alcohol intake, hepatitis B or C, viruses, autoimmune, hereditary and metabolic causes.

Acute liver failure (ALF) is relatively uncommon and is associated with the development of hepatic encephalopathy (confusion, stupor and coma), jaundice, cerebral edema and decreased production of proteins (such as albumin and blood clotting factors) within four weeks of the first symptoms (such as jaundice) of a liver problem. The term fulminant hepatic failure (FHF) is often used synonymously, however it has been proposed that the term hyperacute, acute and subacute liver failure should be used instead. "Hyperacute" liver failure is said to be present if the interval between the onset of jaundice and encephalopathy is less than 7 days. However, this has not received universal acceptance.

Acute liver failure without preexisting liver disease can occur as a result of drug reaction, toxins or viral infection.

Liver failure can also occur as an acute decompensation of chronic liver disease. The triggering factor of decompensation is commonly a viral or bacterial infection or upper gastrointestinal bleeding. Their presentation is similar to acute liver failure.

End stage decompensation of chronic liver failure represents an irreversible deterioration of liver cells. The residual function left is not compatible with life and liver transplantation is the only viable treatment option. However in acute decompensation of chronic liver disease, the function of the remaining viable liver tissue mass may be adequate to maintain homeostasis if the precipitating agent is removed.

Liver dysfunction is also a common consequence of critical illness. In hemodynamically unstable patients, it is often seen as ischemic hepatitis due to inadequate perfusion or as a part of multiple organ dysfunction. Given the number of drugs that the critically-ill patients receive the possibility of drug interaction and toxicity producing liver injury should be borne in mind.

Diagnosis

The consequences of liver failure manifest as a syndrome of metabolic encephalopathy (HE), hepatorenal syndrome, esophageal and gastric varices, ascitis, jaundice, hemodynamic instability, susceptibility to infections and metabolic derangements.

Management

The management of ALF in the ICU setting is discussed below, focusing on each of the systems affected.

Neurological

Cerebral Edema

Acute hepatic damage prevents the liver from metabolizing ammonia, a by-product of normal protein metabolism, to the less-toxic compound urea. In ALF arterial ammonia levels are grossly elevated and an alternative pathway is used for ammonia detoxification. Glutamine synthase metabolizes urea back to glutamine and this results in increased accumulation of glutamine within the brain. The brain cells or astrocytes swell up secondary to this effect leading to cerebral edema and intracranial hypertension.

This is the most accepted hypothesis for the pathogenesis of cerebral edema, although it is regarded as a multifactorial in origin. Ammonia levels are regarded as prognostic marker in ALF.

In management the measures include:

- Elevate head to 30 degrees to facilitate venous drainage
- Appropriate sedation to prevent stimuli from rising intracranial pressure (ICP)
- Avoid hypotension if necessary by use of vasopressors
- Prevent hypoxemia by instituting mechanical ventilation
- Target $PaCO_2$ 35–37 mm Hg (low normal range)
- Tight glycemic control with blood glucose target between 90–110 mg/dL.

Mannitol (0.25–0.5 g/kg) is used to treat intracranial hypertension associated with cerebral edema. However, mannitol is associated with marked reductions in blood pressure through decreases in systemic vascular resistance (SVR) and osmotic diuresis. Boluses of hypertonic saline can be utilized with similar benefits, without the hemodynamic side effects. Doses of 1–2 mL/kg of 3% saline may be given, ideally via a central line, targeting a serum sodium concentration of between 145–155 mmol/L.

Hepatic Encephalopathy

As the clinical course of ALF progresses, hepatic encephalopathy becomes the predominant feature caused by the livers inability to remove toxic substances from the body. Hepatic encephalopathy is a clinical diagnosis and is graded as shown in Table 1.

It is generally accepted that all patients in grade 3 encephalopathy or above will require mechanical ventilation for airway protection. Mechanical ventilation facilitates the use of sedation and analgesia that can reduce cerebral metabolic demand and cerebral blood flow as well as minimizing intracranial pressure rises associated with agitation. Head imaging with

Table 1: Grading of hepatic encephalopathy

Grade	*Level of consciousness*	*Personality and intellect*	*Neurologic signs*	*Electroencephalogram abnormalities*
0	Normal	Normal	Normal	None
1	Trivial lack of awareness; shortened attention span;	None	Subclinical	Normal
2	Lethargy or apathy; disorientation; mild confusion	Restlessness, forgetfulness, agitation	inappropriate behavior; slurred speech; obvious asterixis	Triphasic waves (5 Hz)
3	Somnolence	unable to perform mental tasks; disorientation about time and place	marked confusion; amnesia; occasional fits of rage	Triphasic waves (5 Hz)
4	Coma	None	Decerebration	Delta/slow wave activity

computerized tomography (CT) is used to exclude other causes of decline in mental status, such as intracranial hemorrhage.

Intracranial Pressure Monitoring

The role of ICP monitoring in ALF is controversial. Although such devices allow titration of inotropic support to maintain desirable cerebral perfusion pressures (CPP), the benefits need to be weighed against the risks of their use in the presence of coagulopathy.

Respiratory Compromise

Patients with liver failure may have poor gas exchange, fluctuating level of consciousness that requires intubation and hepatopulmonary syndrome (HPS). HPS is found in 15–20% of patients with cirrhosis due to pulmonary vascular dilation producing arteriovenous shunting. Other factors like pleural effusion and severe ascites may also impair ventilation. High levels of positive end expiratory pressure (PEEP) should be avoided if possible because they may increase hepatic venous pressure and ICP.

Cardiovascular

Hemodynamic derangements consistent with multiple organ failure occur in ALF. Hypotension (systolic, <80 mm Hg) may be present in 15% of patients. Reduced systemic vascular resistance is characteristic in ALF. This may result in hepatic hypoperfusion despite a sometimes elevated cardiac output. These changes are confounded by poor lactate clearance due to hepatic impairment to cause profound hyperlactatemia.

Most patients will require fluid resuscitation on admission. Intravascular volume deficits may be present on admission due to decreased oral intake or GI blood loss. Hemodynamic derangement resembles that of sepsis or cirrhosis with hepatorenal syndrome (low SVR with normal or increased cardiac output). An arterial line should be placed for continuous blood pressure monitoring.

Renal

Acute kidney injury (AKI) is common in the setting of ALF. AKI can be secondary to direct nephrotoxic effects of drugs, raised intra-abdominal pressure, hepatorenal syndrome and acute tubular necrosis (ATN) due to profound hypovolemia and hypotension.

Renal replacement therapy (RRT) should be provided early in the course of AKI complicating ALF to prevent worsening acidosis and fluid overload. Continuous venovenous hemodialysis (CVVHD) is preferred over intermittent hemodialysis to avoid hemodynamic instability.

Hepatorenal Syndrome

Although generally a feature of liver cirrhosis, a rapidly progressive form is commonly seen in the context of ALF. The progressive rise in cardiac output and reduction in SVR results in reduced total vascular resistance and, ultimately, a decline in renal perfusion. The end result is reduced glomerular filtration rate (GFR) and sodium excretion. The pathological basis for this phenomenon is thought to be associated with the accumulation of vasoactive substances such as endotoxin, which are usually cleared by the liver.

Coagulation

The liver synthesises all the coagulation factors apart from factor VIII. Abnormal synthesis of these factors in addition to deficient protein C and antithrombin III and coexistent sepsis mean that severe coagulopathy and low grade DIC are common in ALF. However, clinically significant bleeding is uncommon. The routine use of fresh frozen plasma (FFP) to correct coagulopathies is not recommended. FFP will mask the trends in the prothrombin time that can be used as a prognostic marker. It can also potentiate cerebral edema through increases in intravascular volume. Thrombocytopenia should also not be routinely corrected.

The obvious exception to the rule is the administration of such products in patients who are actively bleeding or before doing invasive procedures such as central line insertion.

Managing poisonings (e.g. acetaminophen, mushroom) requires specific treatment distinct from other, more general issues related to FHF.

Treat acetaminophen (paracetamol, APAP) overdose with N-Acetyl Cysteine (NAC). Researchers theorize that this antidote works by a number of protective mechanisms. It increases glutathione stores, combines directly with NAPQI (metabolite of paracetamol) as a glutathione substitute, and enhances sulfate conjugation. NAC also functions as an antioxidant and has positive inotropic and vasodilating effects, which improve microcirculatory blood flow and oxygen delivery to tissues. These latter effects decrease morbidity and mortality once hepatotoxicity is well established.

Nutrition

Nutritional support should be started as soon as possible. Enteral and parenteral routes are both accepted methods of delivery. Protein intake should not be restricted and dietary laxatives (e.g. lactulose) should be administered to speed the evacuation of nitrogenous waste. The hepatic glycogen stores are exhausted due to decreased gluconeogenesis and hyperinsulinemia, hypoglycemia is commonly seen in liver failure. Infusion of 10% dextrose solutions may be required, at least until feeding is established.

Infection

These patients are prone to infection from Gram negative and Gram positive bacteria and fungi. However, the role of prophylactic antimicrobial drugs is controversial. It is important to implement strict infection control measures, have a high index of suspicion of infection and use appropriate antimicrobial agents early.

The normal systemic features of infection may be absent in patients with ALF and therefore extra vigilance is required. Patients being considered for liver transplantation may benefit from prophylactic antibiotics because sepsis can prevent the proposed procedure.

Consultations

Managing FHF is a team effort. Consultations in the areas of intensive care, gastroenterology, infectious diseases, hematology, neurology, neurosurgery, and transplantation surgery may be needed to address the myriad complex issues that can confront the medical staff.

Liver Transplantation

Detailed analysis of liver transplantation is beyond the scope of this chapter. However it remains the only effective therapy for ALF patients who fail to recover spontaneously. There have been large studies on ALF patients but no single predictive scoring system has been successfully derived due to the wide variety of etiologies. However, the Kings College Hospital Criteria (Table 2) is probably the most widely used with the most diagnostic accuracy.

Contraindications to liver transplantation include irreversible brain damage, accelerating inotrope requirements, uncontrolled sepsis and severe respiratory failure.

Table 2: Kings College Hospital criteria for liver transplantation in acute liver failure

Paracetamol (acetaminophen) overdose	*Non-paracetamol etiology*
• pH <7.3 (irrespective of encephalopathy) Or • All of the following: – Grade III—IV encephalopathy – Creatinine >300 umol/L – Prothrombin time >100 seconds (INR >6.5)	• Prothrombin time >100 seconds Or • Any 3 of the following: – Age <10 years or >40 years – Prothrombin time >50 seconds – Bilirubin >300 umol/L – Time from jaundice to encephalopathy >2 days – Non–A, non–B hepatitis, halothane or drug-induced acute liver failure

22
CHAPTER

Acute Renal Failure in Intensive Care Unit and Renal Replacement Therapy

Pradeep D'Costa

INTRODUCTION

Acute renal failure (ARF) with the concomitant need for renal replacement therapy (RRT) is a common complication in critical care medicine that is still associated with high mortality.

ARF is reported to occur in 20–25% of ICU population, much higher than other hospitalized patients. It often forms a part of the multiple organ dysfunction syndrome caused by sepsis, trauma, severe pneumonia or cardiac failure. ICU patients needing renal replacement therapy have poorer outcomes. ARF represents an independent risk factor for outcome in critically-ill patients. In addition, the early initiation of RRT with adequate doses is associated with improved survival. Therefore, the "under treatment" of ARF should be avoided, and renal replacement therapy should be instituted as soon as the patient fulfils the criteria.

Acute tubular necrosis (ATN) is a broad term used to describe renal failure secondary to various insults which may be nephrotoxic and/or ischemic in origin. However all insults may not be strictly ischemic or nephrotoxic, so a new consensus definition has been established. This approach describes staging of renal failure and puts forward the concept of acute kidney injury. The pathophysiology, definition and diagnosis of ARF are outside the purview of this article.

ARF—PREVENTION AND EARLY RECOGNITION

Clinical Assessment

Detailed history would give information about preexisting conditions such as diabetes and hypertension who are prone to have renal dysfunction. Patients admitted to ICU with life-threatening infections and septic shock are highly likely to develop renal failure. Nurses in ICU who measure urine output hourly readily recognize a key sign of impending renal failure.

Volume Status and ARF

Volume depletion is a well-known precipitating factor for ARF. While it is generally accepted that maintenance of adequate intravascular volume is important, the type and volume of fluid has been the subject of controversy. Hydration has been suggested to prevent renal failure in contrast-induced nephropathy, postcardiac surgery and in drug-induced nephropathy. Over hydration as evidenced by pulmonary edema has to be avoided. So the maintenance of an adequate intravascular volume is an ongoing process requiring multiple assessment and multiple fluid boluses.

Preventing Further Injury

Again ARF is not a single event in time and there can be multiple events, which can compromise kidney function during a single ICU stay. Patients with ATN are highly susceptible to recurrent ischemic damage which may be due to hypotension caused by hypovolemia, dialysis, sepsis, cardiac dysfunction, anesthesia and drugs such as ACE inhibitors. Fluid shifts due to third spacing; decreased perfusion due to cardiac and pulmonary dysfunction can compromise intravascular volume. Renal blood flow may be critically low in patients with heart or liver failure. Therefore, it is important that multiple assessment, and if mandated multiple interventions are necessary to optimize intravascular volume. The level of blood pressure needed to maintain renal blood flow is not very well described. While a mean arterial pressure (MAP) of 65–70 mm of Hg is described as adequate it is obvious that in the elderly hypertensives, diabetics or those with generalized atherosclerosis this level of MAP may result in serious under perfusion.

(i) Dopamine is physiologically appealing as there is an increase in renal blood flow at lower doses. However a large randomized control trial and a rigorous meta-analysis has not supported the use of dopamine.

(ii) Loop diuretics: The conversion of oliguric to nonoliguric ARF, and the flushing out of debris from the tubules are among the many reasons proposed to support the use of loop diuretics in ARF. Even though popular and widely used in varying doses there is no evidence supporting the use of loop diuretics in ARF. A recent review has shown that the use of loop diuretics may be associated with increased mortality even though the number of dialysis required and the oliguric period is decreased.

Avoidance of Nephrotoxins

Every attempt must be made to avoid exposure to nephrotoxins in the critically ill. Normal regulation of renal blood flow can be blocked by nonsteroid anti-inflammatory drugs (NSAIDs), ACE inhibitors or angiotensin receptor blockers. Aminoglycosides are another class of drugs which are commonly used in ICU and a once daily dose of aminoglycosides has been shown to be equally effective but less nephrotoxic in number of studies.

Prophylactic Therapies

N-Acetylcysteine (NAC) has been used as an antioxidant to prevent ARF and the progression of ARF in patients exposed to contrast media. In patients with a high risk of ARF, with background renal dysfunction undergoing radiological interventions involving the use of radiocontrast agents, NAC definitely has a role to play.

Despite meticulous attention to all these patients may develop severe metabolic acidosis (pH <7.1) and hyperkalemia (K^+ >6.0) or fluid overload pulmonary edema. These are indications to commence renal replacement therapy immediately. Early nephrology consultation has been recommended as a method to improve outcomes in ARF. However whether this can be generalized to patients who are in ICUs being looked after by intensivists who are familiar with ARF is unclear. It is more likely that patients in ICU who develop ARF or at risk of ARF will get recognized earlier and will get appropriate treatment with timely nephrology consultation.

Renal Replacement Therapy

Different RRT strategies, like intermittent hemodialysis, continuous venovenous hemofiltration, or hybrid forms that combine the advantages of both techniques are available. Since a general survival benefit has not been demonstrated for either method, it is the task of the nephrologists or intensivist to choose the RRT strategy that is most advantageous for each individual patient. The underlying disease, its severity and stage, the etiology of ARF, the clinical and homodynamic status of the patient, the resources available, and the different costs of therapy may all influence the choice of the RRT strategy.

The indication for initiation and continuation of dialysis are well described. Numerous trials have been published comparing intermittent and continuous modes of renal replacement therapy (RRT). In the Indian scenario, what is likely to determine the mode of RRT will be the economic implications. Continuous techniques are costlier and more demanding on personnel and equipment, albeit more widely applicable in the ICU. A review of RRT has suggested that intermittent RRT is comparable if strict attention is paid to the hemodynamics, prolonging duration and prevention of cooling of dialysate. What may be more important is the experience of the ICU and the volumes of the patients seen rather than a dogmatic approach favoring one or the other techniques.

8

Section

Miscellaneous

SECTION EDITOR: Prakash Shastri

23
CHAPTER

Sampling for Investigations in Critically-ill Patients

Shilpi Khanna

INTRODUCTION

Proper handling of specimens is crucial for obtaining timely and relevant microbiological test results. Specimens submitted for microbiological testing require proper handling from the time of collection through all stages of transport, storage, and processing.

The purpose of this chapter is to review methods of specimen handling, particularly specimen collection, that can be used to modify traditional practices in clinical microbiology.

Collection of specimens for culture differs in two ways from collection of specimens for routine analysis:

- Prevention of contamination by the organisms on the skin is essential if misleading results resulting from growth of contaminants or normal microbiota is to be avoided.
- Proper and prompt transportation to the laboratory is essential to avoid drying of the specimen as well as recovery of the pathogenic organisms which are much delicate than the normal microbial flora.
- The probability of obtaining a "positive" culture increases in proportion to the size of the sample obtained. Sub-optimal samples, whether for blood culture, throat swab or other samples may provide false negative results.

Tenets of Specimen Management

There are some strategic tenets of specimen management and testing in microbiology that stand as standards of care. These set the microbiology specialty apart from other specialities like biochemistry or hematology.

- Universal precautions using gloves, mask and gown need to be taken at all times of sample collection considering all patients as infectious.
- Sample collection guidelines issued by the laboratory should be consulted at all times and whenever required.
- Poor quality specimens must be rejected. Examples of specimen rejection list followed by microbiology laboratories have been listed in Box 1 and Table 1.

Box 1: Specimen rejection criteria used by microbiology laboratory

Clerical errors
Discrepancy between patient identification on requisition and specimen container label
No identification and bar code on the container
General collection and transportation errors
Specimens received in fixative (formalin): Exception, stool for parasites and ova
Foley's catheter/Endotracheal tube tips
Improper or nonsterile container
Leaking container
Dry swab/only one swab for multiple tests
Insufficient sample amount submitted with multiple requests for various organisms
Prolonged transport/improper storage temperature
Saliva instead of sputum specimen
Specimens not appropriate for particular test requested

Table 1: Acceptability and rejection criteria for anaerobic cultures

Acceptable specimens	*Unacceptable specimens*
• Normal sterile body fluids: Bile, pleural, sinus, joint, pericardial and peritoneal fluid, blood. • Surgical specimens from normally sterile sites: Abscess contents, deep aspiration tissue from wounds, sinus. • Suprapubic urine, transtracheal and culdoscopy aspirates • Bone marrow • Uterine contents, if collected using a protected swab	• Saliva, throat swab • Expectorated sputum, endotracheal aspirates • Unprotected bronchoalveolar lavage (BAL) • Vaginal/cervical swab • Feces (except for *Clostridium difficile*) • Colostomy or ileostomy effluent • Skin swabs • Superficial wound swabs • Rectal swab • Urethral swab • Voided/catheterized urine • Semen/prostatic secretions

- Tissue, aspirates, and fluids are always preferable than swabs for culture. While swabs are convenient and easy to use they might pick up extraneous microbes, hold extremely small volumes of the specimen (0.05 mL), make it difficult to get bacteria or fungi away from the swab fibers and onto the media.
- A specimen should be collected prior to administration of antibiotics. Once antibiotics have been started, the flora changes, leading to potentially misleading culture results. If the patient is on antibiotics, samples should be collected at the trough levels or just before the next dose of antibiotics.
- Collect specimens from anatomic sites most likely to yield pathogens and least likely to yield contaminants.
- Adequate volume of the specimen is very important for maximum recovery of pathogens and also to perform

multiple tests on the same specimen. Inadequate volume may lead to false negative results.

- All specimens should be properly labeled to ensure that an accurate diagnosis is being reported on the correct patient. The label should consist of the following parameters.

Patient's full name (not a nickname) Medical record number or other unique identifier (ID) Date and, if appropriate, time when specimen was obtained Specimen source Signature/ initials of collector The label should be affixed directly to the specimen container and not the bag
Bar-coded pre-printed labels with accession numbers generated by an information system may be used.

- Specimen requisition forms or computerized order entry systems should include all important information as
  - Specific site(s) from which specimens were collected;
  - Whether the patient was receiving antimicrobial therapy prior to specimen collection or at the time specimens were collected;
  - Specific pathogens that are being sought;
  - The methods by which specimens were collected; and
  - Whether the patient may be infected with pathogens known to be hazardous to laboratory personnel (e.g. *Brucella* or *Mycobacterium tuberculosis)*
  - A brief clinical history of the patient's illness.

  Such information is necessary to ensure that specimens are processed promptly, that appropriate cultures are performed, that test processing is appropriate for the method of specimen collection (e.g. urine obtained via suprapubic aspiration vs. the clean catch method), and that laboratory personnel are not inadvertently and unknowingly exposed to highly pathogenic microorganisms.

Transportation and Storage of Specimens

In general, specimens collected for microbiological testing should be transported in sterile containers and as promptly as possible for processing. Maybe if delay is inevitable, use of a transport media is used to optimize testing. For health care systems with off-site facilities, transportation procedures should be developed to minimize delays, prevent damage to specimens during transport, and prevent loss of specimens. Needle transport is very unsafe because there is always the risk of a needle stick injury, and syringe transport poses a risk because specimen may be expelled during transport, creating a threat to personnel and environment. Thus, transportation in such a way should be minimized.

Most specimens requiring prolonged storage before processing should be refrigerated at 2–8°C. Refrigeration maintains the viability of pathogens and preserves them in their relative proportions. The latter factor is crucial when semi-quantitative cultures or quantitative cultures (e.g. cultures of respiratory samples or urine) are necessary for interpretation of results. However, blood samples for culture, Cerebrospinal fluid (CSF), genital specimens, eye and internal ear specimens should be transported at room temperature as they might harbor delicate organisms which can die at refrigerating temperatures. For anaerobic cultures specimens need to be transported within 20–30 minutes in anaerobic culture media. Prompt transport of amoebic aspirates is also essential to prevent dying of the delicate trophozoites of *Entamoeba histolytica* if present.

Representative Samples from Critically ill Patients

Sampling sites include those suspected clinically of harboring infection, or if a specific site cannot be identified clinically, blood, urine, and sputum samples are sent. Samples should be sent to the laboratory promptly to allow early incubation and to prevent potentially misleading growth. Swabs if at all collected must be sent in the appropriate transport media.

Blood Culture

Accurate and timely detection of bacteremia and fungemia remains one of the most important functions of clinical microbiology laboratories. Blood culture contamination rates can be minimized by strict adherence to aseptic collection technique. The positive blood culture either establishes or confirms that there is an infectious etiology for the patient's illness. Besides being diagnostic it also has a prognostic value.

Timing of Blood Cultures

Blood cultures should be obtained simultaneously. Drawing blood at intervals is only indicated when it is necessary to document continuous bacteremia in patients with suspected infective endocarditis or other endovascular infections.

Number of Blood Cultures

It has been shown previously that the cumulative yield of pathogens from 3 blood cultures approaches 96% as compared to 80% and 65% with two or single blood cultures respectively. It is thus recommended to collect two to three sets per episode. This practice results in adequate volume of blood cultured and it also helps in identifying contaminants from pathogens. Surveillance blood cultures advocated as a means to allow earlier detection of sepsis are helpful but they add substantial costs to the patient.

Volume of Blood for Culture

The yield of pathogens increases in direct proportion to the volume of blood cultured. For adults, the recommended volumes for blood cultures are 20 to 30 mL per culture. For infants and younger children, the volume of blood drawn should be not more than 1% of the total blood volume.

Distribution of Blood between Aerobic and Anaerobic Blood Culture Bottles

It is recommended that routine blood cultures include paired aerobic/anaerobic blood culture bottles. Blood should always be inoculated in the aerobic bottle first followed by anaerobic bottle in case the recommended blood volume is not collected.

Disinfection of Skin for Blood Culture Collection

To avoid contamination the skin should be cleaned with 70% isopropyl alcohol and allowed to dry thoroughly before venipuncture. Tincture of iodine and chlorhexidine gluconate are superior to povidone-iodine preparations. However, tincture of iodine and chlorhexidine gluconate are equivalent to each other. A contact time of 30 seconds for tincture of iodine and 1.5 to 2 minutes for iodophores is required for complete disinfection. Chlorhexidine gluconate requires the same amount of time as tincture of iodine, but is not associated with allergic reactions and does not need to be cleared off skin after the venipuncture is completed. However, it cannot be used in infants less than 2 months of age.

Blood Culture Collection

Blood for culture should be drawn from veins and not arteries. Blood cultures obtained from indwelling vascular devices are associated with greater contamination rates than those obtained by venipuncture, so should always be paired with another one obtained by venipuncture to assist in interpretation, in the event of a positive result.

After identifying the venipuncture site the rubber septum on the blood culture bottle or tube should be disinfected with 70% isopropyl alcohol and allowed to dry. The skin should then be disinfected for the recommended amount of time. Do not palpate the vein after disinfection of skin. It is recommended that blood be drawn directly into a sterile syringe and then transferred to the blood culture bottle or tube. Drawing blood directly into blood culture vials or bottles is not recommended because of the danger of reflux of the media back into the vein and also that the volume of blood drawn cannot be controlled. After collection, the samples should be transported to the laboratory within two hours. In case of a delay, they should be placed at room temperature for no more than few hours, else kept in an incubator at 37°C.

Urine

Proper collection of urine specimens is vital for accurate results. Contaminated urine submitted for culture wastes time, money and can be clinically misleading. The following steps need be followed for collection of ***midstream clean catch*** early morning specimens of urine.

Males

- Cleanse the penis and retract the foreskin if the patient is not circumcised. Wash with soapy water or pads soaked with liquid soap.
- To minimize contamination with skin flora, keep the foreskin retracted and instruct patient to begin voiding. Discard the first few milliliters of urine, then pass the sterile container into the urine stream and remove before void ends.

Females

- Cleanse the urethral opening and the vaginal vestibule with soapy water or pads soaked with liquid soap, using front-to-back strokes.
- To collect midstream urine, hold the labia apart and instruct patient to begin voiding. Discard the first few milliliters of urine, then pass the sterile container into the urine stream and remove before the void ends.

Straight catheter specimens are usually obtained from the critically ill patients. They are performed when results from clean catch specimens are suspect and diagnosis is critical especially in children and neonates.

- After thoroughly cleaning the urethral and/or vaginal area, and using sterile technique, insert a catheter into the patient's bladder.
- Discard the initial 15–30 mL of urine. Collect and submit sample in a sterile container from the mid-or-later flow of urine.

For catheterized patients, the sampling site should be pre-prepared as aseptically as possible maintaining a sterile, closed catheter system at all times.

- Urine specimens should he obtained aseptically without opening the catheter-collection junction.
- Clean the catheter port thoroughly with 70% alcohol, allow it to dry.
- Urine should be aspirated from the distal end of the catheter with sterile needle and syringe after disinfecting the area.
- Transfer to a sterile container.
- Never submit urine for culture from the catheter collection bag.
- Three consecutive first morning whole urine specimens (not less than 100 mL) are recommended for mycobacterial culture.
- Do not submit 24-hour urine collections for culture.

Suprapubic aspirates should be clearly labeled. The specimen should be sent to the laboratory immediately within 2 hours and examined microscopically for organisms, casts and crystals. 24 hours urine collections and Foley's catheter tips are not recommended for culture.

The recommended volumes of urine samples for various cultures are as follows:

- Bacterial culture (0.5–1 mL)
- Fungal culture (>20 mL)
- Mycobacterial culture (100 mL)
- Viral culture or tests (10–50 mL).

In the laboratory, urine is plated on to culture medium with a calibrated loop and incubated for 18—24 hours prior to examination. For midstream urine specimen significant pyuria refers to ≥10 pus cells/high power field in an uncentrifuged sample in patients who are not neutropenic. Significant bacteriuria refers to ≥10^5 cfu/mL in immunocompetent patients not on antibiotics; lower counts may be significant in nosocomial infection or patients on antibiotics. All catheters specimens show bacterial growth if the catheter has been in place for more than 2 days. Isolation of the same organism from blood confirms a significant culture.

Respiratory Samples

Upper respiratory tract samples usually include specimens from the ears, the mucus membranes lining the nose and throat above the epiglottis, and the sinuses.

- *Throat swabs:* Throat specimens require a firm, thorough sampling of the throat and tonsils, avoiding cheeks, gums, and teeth. Do not obtain throat sample if epiglottis is inflamed, as sampling may cause serious respiratory obstruction. Depress tongue gently with a tongue depressor and extend sterile swab between the tonsillar pillars and behind the uvula and sweep the swab back and forth across the posterior pharynx, tonsillar areas and any inflamed or ulcerated areas to obtain sample. *Haemophilus influenzae, Staphylococcus aureus, Neisseria meningitidis,* and *Streptococcus pneumoniae* are not etiologic agents of pharyngitis and should not be sought in throat cultures.
- *Aspirates from sinuses:* Swabs are not recommended for otitis media or sinusitis. An aspirate should be submitted for culture. Most cases of otitis media can be diagnosed clinically and treated without culture support.
- *Nasal swabs:* They are submitted primarily for the detection of staphylococcal carriers. Insert a sterile swab into the nose until resistance is met at the level of the turbinates (approximately 1 inch into the nose). Rotate the swab against the nasal mucosa and repeat the process on the other side.
- *Nasopharyngeal suction:* Submitted for the detection of carriers of *S. pyogenes, N. meningitidis, C. diphtheriae* and *B. pertussis.*
- *Nasopharyngeal swabs:* Submitted primarily for the detection of *N. meningitidis* and to diagnose *B. pertussis.*
- *Oral cultures:* Used to prepare smears for the detection of yeast or fusospirochaetal disease.

Lower respiratory tract samples are the best indicator of pneumonia, bronchitis, bronchiolitis and pleural space infections. The key points to be remembered when obtaining specimens for the diagnosis of respiratory infections.

- *First morning sputum* is always best for culture. If sputum cultures are ordered thrice, it is best to collect three early morning samples on three consecutive days. Do not have the patient expectorate saliva or postnasal drip into the container. Place specimen in sterile screw-cap container. Refrigerate specimen for transport. Deliver to laboratory as soon as possible. Presence of more than 10 squamous epithelial cells/low power field is indicative of a poor quality specimen and in such cases a fresh specimen of sputum should be submitted for examination.
- *Blood cultures* that accompany sputum specimens may occasionally be helpful, particularly in high-risk community acquired pneumonia patients.
- The laboratory should be contacted for specific instructions prior to collection of specimens for fastidious pathogens such as *Bordetella pertussis.*
- *Tracheostomy and endotracheal aspirations:* Suction specimens from intubated patients can be taken by sterile suction catheters into a sterile suction trap. Tracheostomy tube tip or endotracheal tube tip are not recommended for culture, hence are not accepted.
- *Bronchoscopy specimens:* These include bronchoalveolar lavage, bronchial washing, bronchial brushing and trans-bronchial biopsy specimens. These samples are collected by the clinicians and sent to the laboratory in sterile containers.
- *Fungal cultures:* Recommended volume of the samples is 3–5 mL. Collect three early morning fresh specimens resulting from deep cough or sputum induction. Lung biopsy specimens or lung aspirates are also appropriate.
- *Mycobacterial cultures:* Recommended volume of the samples for mycobacterial cultures is 5–10 mL. Collect three early morning fresh specimens resulting from deep cough or sputum induction. Bronchial aspirates, lung biopsy specimens or lung aspirates are also appropriate.
- *Pneumocystis spp.*: Use induced sputum, bronchoalveolar lavage or lung biopsy specimen.
- Calcium alginate swabs are not acceptable for nucleic acid amplification testing.

Pus Samples, Wound Swabs, Tissue Samples

- *Aspirated pus* must be sent to the laboratory immediately or a swab sample may be taken and sent in transport medium. Pus is preferable for bacterial isolation.
- *Fungal examinations of superficial lesions:* Clean the surface with 70% alcohol. Using a blade, scrape the periphery of

the lesion border. Samples from scalp hair lesions should include hair that is selectively collected for examination. If there is nail involvement, obtain scrapings of debris or material beneath the nail plate. Transport in folded filter paper or if material is very scanty, put it directly on a glass slide, put a drop of potassium hydroxide over it and put a coverslip and send it to the laboratory.

- *Tissue samples* for culture should always be sent in sterile containers without any fixative.

Sterile Body Fluids and Cerebrospinal Fluid

The prompt, accurate diagnosis of bacterial meningitis is among the most important tasks confronting laboratories. Strict aseptic techniques must be followed while collecting cerebrospinal fluid (CSF), both to minimize specimen contamination and to prevent introduction of bacteria into the central nervous system. The risk of contamination is low when the skin is adequately disinfected using either an iodophore or chlorhexidine prior to lumbar puncture. CSF specimens should be transported immediately to the laboratory. From collection through processing, CSF specimens (except aliquots collected for viral cultures) should not be refrigerated until initial processing is completed. Attempt to collect as much sample as possible for multiple tests (minimum recommended is 1 mL). Multiple test requests on small volume samples should be prioritized.

For other body fluids as ascetic, pleural, peritoneal, pericardial fluids, maximum possible volume of specimens should be sent for examination. Interpretation of culture results from drains that have been in place for more than 3 days may be difficult due to the presence of colonizing bacteria and yeast and should therefore not be attempted.

Gastrointestinal Samples

Gastrointestinal (GI) infections include a wide variety of disease presentations as well as infectious agents. The gastrointestinal tract includes the esophagus, stomach, duodenum, small intestine and colon. The specimen of choice to diagnose diarrheal illness is the diarrheal stool, not a formed stool or a swab.

i. *Stool specimens:* Keep the stool specimens cool, do not incubate them. If the sample cannot be plated within 1 hour of collection, it should be mixed with transport medium. Either ask the patient to pass stool directly into a sterile wide mouthed, leak-proof container with a tight fitting lid or ask him to pass stool into a clean, dry bedpan and then to transfer it into a sterile leak-proof container with a tight fitting lid.

ii. *Rectal swabs:* Submitted primarily for the detection of *N. gonorrhoeae, Shigella species* and anal carriage of *Streptococcus pyogenes* and vancomycin-resistant enterococci (VRE).
iii. *Gastric lavage:* Submitted primarily for the detection of *M. tuberculosis* in patients (most frequently children) unable to produce quality sputum. Should be performed after the patient wakes in the morning so that sputum swallowed during sleep is still in the stomach.
iv. Toxin or nucleic acid amplification testing for *C. difficile* should only be done on diarrheal stool, not formed stools, unless the physician notes that the patient has ileus.

Serologic Diagnosis of Infectious Diseases

For most diseases, serological testing is not a surrogate for culture or other diagnostic tests. Specimens obtained for serological analysis should be collected either in sterile evacuated tubes or in serum separator tubes. Strict aseptic technique should be used during venipuncture. Adequate volumes of blood should be drawn for anticipated tests. To prevent loss of immunologic reactivity and growth of contaminating microorganisms, specimens should be transported promptly to the laboratory and centrifuged, and the serum should be poured off and refrigerated or frozen immediately.

A clotted blood specimen allows antibodies to viral and atypical agents to be assayed. It is usual to send acute and convalescent sample (14 days) serum to determine increasing antibody titres. Single-sample titres may be used to determine previous exposure and carrier status. Hemolyzed samples are not acceptable for serologic assays.

Antibiotic Assays

Antibiotic assays are usually performed for drugs with a narrow therapeutic range, such as aminoglycosides and vancomycin. Vancomycin trough levels are normally drawn 30 minutes prior to fourth scheduled dose and as clinically required thereafter. Vancomycin peak levels are rarely useful. Aminoglycoside levels can be drawn between 8–24 hours after the first dose and are used to calculate the dosing interval with an aminoglycoside nomogram. Peak levels 30 minutes after infusion may occasionally be useful in calculating peak- to- MIC ratios antibiotic therapeutic levels (Table 2).

Table 2: Trough and peak levels of antibiotics

Antibiotics	*Trough levels (mg/L)*	*Peak levels(mg/L)*
Amikacin	<8	30
Gentamicin	<2	4–10
Tobramycin	<2	4–10
Vancomycin	<20	30–50

FURTHER READING

1. Baron EJ, Miller JM, Weinstein MP, Richter SS, Gilligan PH, Thomson RB Jr, et al. A guide to utilization ofthe microbiology laboratory for diagnosis of infectious diseases:2013 recommendations by the Infectious Diseases Society of America (IDSA) and the American Society for Microbiology (ASM)(a). Clin Infect Dis. 2013; 57(4):e22-e121.
2. Clinical Laboratory Standards Institute. Principles and procedures for blood cultures; Approved Guideline. CLSI document M47-A. Wayne, PA: Clinical and Laboratory Standards Institute, 2007.
3. Cockerill FR 3rd, Wilson JW, Vetter EA, Goodman KM, Torgerson CA, Harmsen WS, et al. Optimal testing parameters for blood cultures. Clin Infect Dis. 2004;38(12):1724-30. Epub 2004 May 25.
4. Isenberg HD, Clinical Microbiology Procedures Handbook. 2nd Edition Update. American Society for Microbiology, Washington DC, 2007.
5. Wilson ML. General principles of specimen collection and transport. Clin Infect Dis. 1996;22(5):766-77.

24

CHAPTER

Needlestick Injury

Lawni Goswami

INTRODUCTION

After performing phlebotomy on a patient with acquired immune deficiency syndrome (AIDS), a nurse sustained a deep needle stick injury. She removed the gloves and washed her hands immediately. She had a negative baseline human immunodeficiency virus (HIV) test and refused zidovudine prophylaxis. Because her patient was not known to have hepatitis C virus (HCV) infection and did not have clinical evidence of liver disease, the nurse did not receive baseline testing for exposure to HCV. Eight months after the incident, she was hospitalized with acute hepatitis. She was found to be seropositive for HIV nine months after the incident. Sixteen months after the incident, she tested positive for anti-HCV antibodies and was diagnosed with chronic HCV infection. Her clinical condition continued to deteriorate, and she died 28 months after the needlestick injury.

Needlestick injuries are wounds caused by needles that accidentally puncture the skin. It is a hazard for people who work with hypodermic syringes and other needle equipment. These injuries can occur at any time when people use, dis assemble, or dispose of needles. When not disposed of properly, needles can become concealed in linen or garbage and injure other workers who encounter them unexpectedly. These injuries transmit infectious diseases, especially blood-borne viruses. Concern includes the HIV which leads to AIDS, hepatitis B, and hepatitis C.

EPIDEMIOLOGY

The average risk following percutaneous exposure to HIV-infected blood in health care settings is about 3 per 1,000 injuries, less than 1:1000 following mucocutaneous exposure, and has never been recorded following contact of HIV blood with intact skin.

Certain features of a percutaneous injury carry a particularly high-risk:

- A deep injury
- Terminal HIV-related illness in the source patient

- Visible blood on the device which caused the injury
- Injury with a needle which had been placed in a source patient's artery or vein.

Prevention of avoidable exposure in an occupational setting: This is of prime importance. The Health Protection Agency advises the following:

GENERAL MEASURES

- Wash hands before and after contact with each patient, and before putting on and after removing gloves.
- Change gloves between patients.
- Cover existing wounds, skin lesions and all breaks in exposed skin with waterproof dressings, wear gloves if hands are extensively affected.
- Wear gloves where contact with blood can be anticipated.
- Avoid sharps usage where possible, and where sharps usage is essential, exercise particular care in handling and disposal.
- Avoid wearing open footwear in situations where blood may be spilt, or where sharp instruments or needles are handled.
- Clear up spillage of blood promptly and disinfect surfaces.
- Pre-employment occupational health assessment should identify those with damaged skin, e.g. fissured hand eczema, who may be at higher risk of occupationally acquired infection, and ensure that advice is given about minimising any occupational health risk to which they may be exposed.
- Wear gloves when cleaning equipment prior to sterilization or disinfection, when handling chemical disinfectant and when cleaning up spillages.
- Follow safe procedures for disposal of contaminated waste.

SPECIFIC MEASURES

This will obviously depend on the procedure being undertaken, but may include:

- Use of new, single-use disposable injection equipment for all injections is highly recommended. Sterilizable injection should only be considered if single use equipment is not available and if the sterility can be documented with time, steam and temperature indicators.
- Discard contaminated sharps immediately and without recapping in puncture and liquid proof containers that are closed, sealed and destroyed before completely full.
- Document the quality of the sterilization for all medical equipment used for percutaneous procedures.
- Wash hands with soap and water before and after procedures; use of protective barriers such as gloves, gowns aprons, masks, goggles for direct contact with blood and other body fluids.

- Disinfect instruments and other contaminated equipment.
- Handle properly soiled linen. (Soiled linen should be handled as little as possible. Gloves and leakproof bags should be used if necessary. Cleaning should occur outside patient areas, using detergent and hot water).

MANAGEMENT

Wash clean wounds/flush mucous membranes immediately (use of caustic agents or squeezing the wound is discouraged; data lacking regarding antiseptics).

Assess risk by doing the following:

Characterize Exposure

Determine/evaluate source of exposure by medical history, risk behavior, and testing for hepatitis B/C, HIV.

Evaluate and test exposed individual for hepatitis B, hepatitis C and HIV.

Follow local or national or international protocol.

First Aid

- Contaminated needle stick, sharps injury, bite or scratch - encourage bleeding, wash with soap and running water.
- Blood or body fluid in eyes or mouth—irrigate with copious quantities of cold water.
- Blood or body fluid on broken skin—encourage bleeding if possible, and wash with soap under running water (but without scrubbing).

Report incident and discuss with local public health consultant immediately.

Investigations

Take blood for virology, (HIV, hepatitis B, hepatitis C) from the injured worker. Start post-exposure prophylaxis (PEP) where appropriate and consider need for antibiotic therapy or hepatitis B immunization.

Documentation

Fill out accident book and complete critical event audit. How can subsequent events be prevented?

Follow-up

Ensure adequate follow up of both care worker and donor. The care worker in particular will require early involvement by the occupation health service. They may need specific advice about having to take sick leave if medication is required, and the possible requirement for psychological support.

Exposure to Hepatitis B

If the health care worker is:

- Not vaccinated: Give HBIG 0.06 mL/kg IM and initiate hepatitis B vaccine

- If vaccinated: Do anti-HBs on exposed person
- If titer ≥10 million IU/mL, no therapy
- If titer <10 million IU/mL, give HBIG + 1 dose HB vaccine.

Exposure to Hepatitis C

Determine antibody to hepatitis C for both exposed person and, if possible, exposure source. If source positive or unknown and exposed person negative, follow-up HCV testing for HCV RNA (detectable in blood in 1–3 weeks) and HCV antibody (90% who seroconvert will do so by 3 months) is advised. Persons who remain viremic 24 weeks after exposure should be treated with a course of targeted direct acting agents after determination of the HCV genotype. Primary (immediate) post-exposure prophylaxis is not recommended. Rather, the HCW should be monitored for evidence of long-term infection with serial HCV RNA determinations. If HCV RNA is detectable >6 months after exposure, treatment with direct acting agents (selected based on the genotype) should be initiated. Case-control study suggested risk factors for occupational HCV transmission include percutaneous exposure to needle that had been in artery or vein, deep injury, male sex of health care worker and was more likely when source viral load >6 log10 copies/mL.

Human Immunodeficiency Virus Post-exposure Prophylaxis

Human immunodeficiency virus (HIV) post-exposure prophylaxis (PEP) should be initiated as soon as possible after exposure (within a few hours). PEP is unlikely to be effective and not recommended more than 72 hours after exposure.

If status of source patient is unknown, and rapid HIV testing is available it is reasonable to await results of this test before starting PEP. Otherwise, therapy should not be delayed pending virologic or serologic confirmation of source patient status. The decision to initiate PEP is a clinical judgment made in concert with the exposed individual and is based on the following factors.

Potentially infectious substances include: blood, unfixed tissues, CSF; semen and vaginal secretions (these have not been implicated in occupational transmission of HIV); synovial, pleural, peritoneal, ascitic, and amniotic fluids; other visibly bloody fluids.

Fluids of low or negligible risk for transmission, unless visibly bloody include: urine, sweat, vomitus, stool, saliva, nasal secretions, tears, and sputum.

Exposure of intact skin: regardless of whether the substance is potentially infectious or not, and regardless of the HIV status of the source patient: PEP is not indicated.

Exposure of mucous membranes (e.g. blood splash to the eye) or non-intact skin (e.g. abraded skin, open wound, dermatitis) or percutaneously (e.g. as a consequence of a needle stick, scalpel, or other sharps injury or cut): PEP may be indicated.

The PEP currently consist of a 28-day course of treatment with a triple combination of antiretroviral drugs, has significant side effects, and needs careful follow up.

25

CHAPTER

Sterilization and Waste Management

Jyoti Randhawa

Management of hospital waste is essential to maintain hygienic, esthetics, cleanliness and control of environmental pollution.

The hospital waste like body parts, organs, tissues, blood and body fluids along with soiled linen, along with used needles, syringes and other sharps are to be properly collected, segregated, stored, transported, treated and disposed of in safe manner to prevent nosocomial or hospital-acquired infection. The biomedical waste scattered in and around the hospitals invites flies, insects, rodents, cats and dogs that are responsible for the spread of communication disease like plague and rabies. Rag pickers in the hospital, sorting out the garbage are at a risk of getting tetanus and HIV infections. It becomes primary responsibility of Health administrators to manage hospital waste in a safe and eco-friendly manner.

CENTRALIZED TREATMENT FACILITY

Under Biomedical Waste (Management and Handling) Rules 1998 updated in 2016, all health care institutions are required to handle biomedical waste in a specified manner. The government hospitals and major private hospitals have their own arrangement for treatment of biomedical waste. The smaller nursing homes and clinics, which cannot make their own arrangements due to high cost involved in treatment facilities, require some alternative modalities. Keeping in view the difficulties faced by smaller nursing homes/clinics/blood banks/diagnostic laboratories, etc. Government is taking initiatives to establish centralized waste treatment facilities.

CLASSIFICATION OF HAZARDOUS WASTE

WHO has classified hazardous waste into following categories:

1. *Infectious waste (suspected to contain pathogens):* Laboratory culture, waste from isolation wards, tissue-swabs, material in contact with infected patient, excreta.
2. *Pathological waste* (containing human tissue or fluids): Body parts, blood and other body fluids, fetuses.

3. *Sharps (Sharp material):* Needles; infusion sets; scalpels; knives; blades; broken glass.
4. *Pharmaceutical waste (containing pharmaceuticals):* Expired drugs; contaminated bottles; boxes.
5. *Genotoxic waste:* Waste containing cytostatic drugs; genotoxic chemicals.
6. *Chemical waste:* Laboratory reagents; film developer expired disinfectants, solvents.
7. *Waste with heavy metals:* Batteries; broken thermometer.
8. *Pressurized containers:* Gas cylinders; gas cartridges; aerosol cans.
9. *Radioactive material:* Unused liquid from radiotherapy; contaminated glass ware; urine excreta from patient treated with unsealed radionucleotides.

Frequently asked Questions Biomedical Waste Management

1. What are biomedical wastes?
Biomedical wastes are defined as waste that is generated during the diagnosis, treatment or immunization of human beings or animals, or in research activities pertaining thereto, or in the production of biologicals.

2. What are biodegradable and nonbiodegradable wastes?
Biodegradable waste means any waste that is capable of undergoing anaerobic or aerobic decomposition, such as food and garden waste, and paper and paperboard. It also includes waste from households, which because of its nature and composition is similar to biodegradable waste from households.

Nonbiodegradable wastes are the wastes that cannot be decomposed by bacteria, e.g. plastics, bottles and tins.

3. What is the quantum of waste that is generated by a hospital?
The quantum of waste that is generated in India is estimated to be 1–2 kg per bed per day in a hospital and 600 g per day per bed in a general practitioner's clinic. For example, a 100 bedded hospital will generate 100–200 kg of hospital waste/day. It is estimated that only 5–10% of this comprises of hazardous/ infectious waste (5–10 kg/day).

4. What are the hazards associated with poor health care waste management?
Proper disposal of biomedical waste is of paramount importance because of its infectious and hazardous characteristics. Improper disposal can result in the following:

- Organic portion ferments and attracts fly breeding
- Injuries from sharps to all categories of health care personnel and waste handlers
- Increase risk of infections to medical, nursing and other hospital staff

Table 1: Persons at risk and mode of transmission

Procedure	*Person at risk*	*Mode of transmission*
Collection of blood samples	Patient health worker	Contaminated needle, gloves, skin puncture by needle or container, contamination of hands by blood
Transfer of specimens (within laboratory)	Laboratory personnel	Contamination of exterior of specimen container, Broken container, splash of specimen
HIV serology and virology	Laboratory personnel	Skin puncture, splash of specimen, Broken specimen container, perforated gloves
Cleaning and maintenance	Laboratory personnel supporting staff	Skin puncture or contamination, splashes, contaminated work surface
Waste disposal	Laboratory personnel support staff transport worker	Contact with contaminated waste, puncture wounds and cuts
Shipment of specimens	Transport worker, postal worker	Broker or leaking specimen, containers and packages

- Injuries from sharps to health workers and waste handlers
- Poor infection control can lead to nosocomial infections in patients particularly HIV, hepatitis B and C.
- Increase in risk associated with hazardous chemicals and drugs being handled by persons handling wastes
- Poor waste management encourages unscrupulous persons to recycle disposables and disposed drugs for repacking and reselling
- Development of resistant strains of microorganisms.

5. Who are the persons at risk of the hazards of medical procedures?

Depending on the type of procedures, the persons at risk and mode of transmission in some common medical procedures are in Table 1:

6. What are the responsibilities of health care institutions regarding biomedical waste management?

It is mandatory for such institutions to:

- Set up biomedical waste treatment facilities like incinerators, autoclave and microwave systems for treatment of the wastes.
- Make an application to the concerned authorities for grant of authorization.
- Submit a report regarding information about the categories and quantities of biomedical wastes handled during the preceding year by 31 January every year.
- Maintain records about the generation, collection, reception, storage, transportation, treatment, disposal and/or any form of handling biomedical waste.
- Report immediately any accident to the prescribed authority.

7. What are the different hospital waste categories?

Table 2: Hospital waste categories

Category	*Type of waste*	*Type of bag or container to be used*	*Treatment and disposal options*
(1)	(2)	(3)	(4)
Yellow	(a) Human anatomical waste: Human tissues, organs, body parts and fetus below the viability period (as per the Medical Termination of Pregnancy Act 1971, amended from time-to-time)	Yellow colored nonchlorinated plastic bags	Incineration or Plasma pyrolysis or deep burial
	(b) Animal anatomical waste: experimental animal carcasses, body parts, organs, tissues, including the waste generated from animals used in experiments or testing in veterinary hospitals or colleges or animal houses		
	(c) Soiled waste: Items contaminated with blood, body fluids like dressings, plaster casts, cotton swabs and bags containing residual or discarded blood and blood components		Incineration or plasma pyrolysis or deep burial. In absence of above facilities, autoclaving or microwaving/hydroclaving followed by shredding or mutilation or combination of sterilization and shredding. Treated waste to be sent for energy recovery
	(d) Expired or Discarded Medicines: Pharmaceutical waste like antibiotics, cytotoxic drugs including all items contaminated with cytotoxic drugs along with glass or plastic ampoules, vials etc.	Yellow coloured nonchlorinated plastic bags or containers	Expired cytotoxic drugs and items contaminated with cytotoxic drugs to be returned back to the manufacturer or supplier for incineration at temperature >1200°C or to common biomedical waste treatment facility or hazardous waste treatment, storage and disposal

Contd...

Contd...

Category	*Type of waste*	*Type of bag or container to be used*	*Treatment and disposal options*
(1)	(2)	(3)	(4)
			facility for incineration at >1200°C or encapsulation or plasma pyrolysis at >1200°C. All other discarded medicines shall be either sent back to manufacturer or disposed by incineration
	(e) Chemical waste: Chemicals used in production of biological and used or discarded disinfectants	Yellow colored containers or non chlorinated plastic bags	Disposed of by incineration or plasma pyrolysis or encapsulation in hazardous waste treatment, storage and disposal facility
	(f) Chemical liquid waste: Liquid waste generated due to use of chemicals in production of biological and used or discarded disinfectants, silver X-ray film developing liquid, discarded formalin, infected secretions, aspirated body fluids, liquid from laboratories and floor washings, cleaning, housekeeping and disinfecting activities, etc.	Separate collection system leading to effluent treatment system	After resource recovery, the chemical liquid waste shall be pretreated before mixing with other waste water. The combined discharge shall conform to the discharge norms given in schedule-III
	(g) Discarded linen, mattresses, beddings contaminated with blood or body fluid	Nonchlorinated yellow plastic bags or suitable packing material	Nonchlorinated chemical disinfection followed by incineration or plasma pyrolysis or for energy recovery. In absence of above facilities, shredding or mutilation or combination of sterilization and shredding. Treated waste to be sent for energy recovery or incineration or plasma pyrolysis

Contd...

Contd...

Category	*Type of waste*	*Type of bag or container to be used*	*Treatment and disposal options*
(1)	(2)	(3)	(4)
	(h) Microbiology, biotechnology and other clinical laboratory waste: Blood bags, laboratory cultures, stocks or specimens of microorganisms, live or attenuated vaccines, human and animal cell cultures used in research, industrial laboratories, production of biological, residual toxins, dishes and devices used for cultures	Autoclave safe plastic bags or containers	Pretreat to sterilize with nonchlorinated chemicals on-site as per National AIDS Control Organization or World Health Organization guidelines thereafter for Incineration
Red	Contaminated waste (Recyclable): Wastes generated from disposable items such as tubing, bottles, intravenous tubes and sets, catheters, urine bags, syringes (without needles and fixed needle syringes) and vacutainers with their needles cut) and gloves	Red colored nonchlorinated plastic bags or containers	Autoclaving or microwaving/ hydroclaving followed by shredding or mutilation or combination of sterilization and shredding. Treated waste to be sent to registered or authorized recyclers or for energy recovery or plastics to diesel or fuel oil or for road making, whichever is possible. Plastic waste should not be sent to landfill sites.
White (Translucent)	Waste sharps including metals: Needles, syringes with fixed needles, needles from needle tip cutter or burner, scalpels, blades, or any other contaminated sharp object that may cause puncture and cuts. This includes both used, discarded and contaminated metal sharps	Puncture proof, leak proof, tamper proof containers	Autoclaving or dry heat sterilization followed by shredding or mutilation or encapsulation in metal container or cement concrete; combination of shredding cum autoclaving; and sent for final disposal to iron foundries (having consent to operate from the State Pollution Control Boards or Pollution Control Committees) or sanitary landfill or designated concrete waste sharp pit

Contd...

Contd...

Category	*Type of waste*	*Type of bag or container to be used*	*Treatment and disposal options*
(1)	(2)	(3)	(4)
Blue	(a) Glassware: Broken or discarded and contaminated glass including medicine vials and ampoules except those contaminated with cytotoxic wastes	Cardboard boxes with blue colored marking	Disinfection (by soaking the washed glass waste after cleaning with detergent and sodium hypochlorite treatment) or through autoclaving or microwaving or hydroclaving and then sent for recycling
	(b) Metallic body implants	Cardboard boxes with blue colored marking	

8. What do the terms disinfection and sterilization actually denote?

Disinfection refers to procedures which reduce the number of microorganisms on an object or surface but not the complete destruction of all microorganism or spores.

Sterilization on the other hand, refers to procedures, which would remove all microorganisms, including spores, from an object. Sterilization is undertaken either by dry heat (for 2 hours at 170°C in an electric oven—method of choice for glass ware and sharps) or by various forms of moist heat (i.e. boiling in water for an effective contact time of 20 minutes or steam sterilization in an autoclave at 15 lb/sq inch at 121°C for 20 min).

9. What are the disinfectants commonly used for disinfection of materials contaminated with blood and body fluids?

The recommended dilutions for these chlorine releasing compounds are given in Table 3.

10. How is disinfection of the various items commonly used in the hospital carried out?

Table 3: Dilutions of disinfectants

Name of disinfectant	*Available chlorine*	*Required chlorine*	*Required chlorine contact period*	*Amount of disinfectant to be dissolved in 1 liter of water*
Sodium hypochlorite	5%	0.5%	30 min	100 mL
Calcium hypochlorite	70%	0.5%	30 min	7.0 g
Na hypochlorite powder	-	0.5%	30 min	8.5 g
Na Dichloroisocyanurate (NaDCC) tablets	60%	0.5%	30 min	4 tablets
Chloramine	25%	0.5%	30 min	20 g

Table 4: Common hospital items and their disinfection

General use items	*Disinfection*
Bed pans, bowls	Wash with hot water and dry disinfect with phenol after use by infected patients autoclave
Crockery, cutlery	Wash with hot water/detergent and keep dry
Floors	Vacuum clean; No use of broom
Furniture	Damp dust with detergent/phenol/2% Lysol
Mattresses/Pillows	Use water impermeable cover Wash cover with detergent and keep dry Disinfect with phenol/2% lysol
Endoscopes/Arthroscopes/Laparoscopes/Fiberoptic endoscopes	Immerse in 2% Cidex solution Use latex gloves, eye protection plastic covering mask while handling
Ambu bags	Ideally heat disinfect Immerse in 2% glutaraldehyde and wash with sterile distilled water to reduce respiratory irritation
Ventilatory circuits	Ethylene oxide sterilization

Table 5: Environment emission standards

Parameters	*Conc mg/N.cu m at 12% CO_2 correction*
Particulate matter	150
Nitrogen oxides	450
HCL	50

11. How long can biomedical waste be stored?

Immediate treatment and disposal are ideal procedures to be followed for disposal of biomedical waste. Untreated biomedical waste however, can be stored for not more than 48 hours. If for some reason, it becomes necessary to store the waste beyond such period, permission from the local state authority must be taken and it must be ensured that it does not adversely affect human health and the environment.

12. What are the emission standards for incineration?

13. What are the standards and requirements for incineration?

- Minimum height of the stack should be 30 meters above the ground
- Above emission limits should be achieved
- Waste to be incinerated not to be disinfected with chlorine substance
- Chlorinated plastics should not be incinerated
- Toxic metals in incineration ash should be limited to within regulatory quantities
- Only low sulfur fuels like LDO/LSHS to be used as fuel
- The common treatment facility (CTF) should be located away from human habitation.

There are three main treatment methods for biomedical waste: steam sterilization, chemical treatment and incineration.

Complete destruction of commercial preparations of bacterial spores is the criterion used to judge effectiveness of various treatments. Some specialized alternative methods also exist, including dry heat, gas sterilization and irradiation.

Steam sterilization, or autoclaving, is the main treatment process for dealing with microbiology wastes. It is also appropriate for sterilizing reusable items. The appearance of waste is not changed by autoclaving, and thus it is not apparent that the waste has been treated. Volume reduction is only 30 percent. Autoclaving is often followed by mechanical shredding to reduce volume and render waste unusable.

Chemical disinfectants such as acids, alkalis, alcohols and hydrogen peroxide can be used to disinfect waste. These destroy microorganisms, but do not affect bacterial spores. They are appropriate for treating liquid waste which is then discharged to sanitary sewers.

When properly operated, *incinerators* kill pathogens, destroy anatomical waste beyond recognition, and render sharps unusable. With effective pollution control devices in place, incineration is now the method of choice for biomedical waste disposal, recommended by the Canadian Standards Association (CSA), the World Health Organization (WHO) and the United States Environmental Protection Agency.

What is the present status of fumigation or fogging?

Fumigation in health care facilities and other related institutions should be limited to those instances where the benefits clearly exceed the risks of human exposure or environmental damage. Decontamination of an unoccupied building following a bioterrorism incident would meet this criterion. In situations where the building is occupied and the potential for recontamination is high, the benefits of fumigation do not appear to exceed the risks. Before potentially risky procedures such as fumigation are considered, simpler and safer approaches such as enhanced cleaning should be considered.

The Ministry of Environment and Forests has come up with New Bio-Medical Waste Management Rules 2016.

The salient features are:

- Vaccination camps, blood donation camps, surgical camps or any other healthcare activity have been included.
- Chlorinated plastic bags, gloves and blood bags to be phased out within two years.
- Biomedical waste to be segregated into 4 categories instead of 10.
- Bar-Code System for bags or containers containing biomedical waste for disposal.
- Pretreatment of the laboratory waste, microbiological waste, blood samples and blood bags through disinfection or sterilization on-site in the manner as prescribed by WHO or NACO.

- Procedure to get authorization simplified. Automatic authorization for bedded hospitals and 1 time authorization for non-bedded HCFs.
- Training and regular immunization to all health care workers.
- All major accidents to be reported.
- Immunize all its health care workers and others involved in handling of biomedical waste for protection against diseases including hepatitis B and tetanus that are likely to be transmitted by handling of biomedical waste.
- State government to provide land for setting up common biomedical waste treatment and disposal facility and no occupier can set up a facility, if a service of common biomedical waste treatment facility is available within 75 km.
- Existing incinerators to achieve the standards for retention time in secondary chamber and dioxin and furans within two years.

26

CHAPTER

Nursing Communication in Intensive Care Units

Anna George, Raymond D Savio

INTRODUCTION

Communication is the art of transmitting information, ideas and attitudes from one person to another. In other words, communication is the process of meaningful interaction between human beings.

One of the main causes of errors in diagnosis or treatment in hospitals is poor communication. Effective communication, which is, accurate, and understood by the recipient, reduces errors and results in improved patient safety.

Clear communication to the patient and family regarding diagnosis, treatment, plan of care, risks, benefits and alternatives of treatment is an important requirement. Moreover, it is actually part of the patient and family's right to know what is going on and participate in the decision process.

The American College of Critical Care Medicine recommends patient-centered care (PCC) practices to improve outcomes in the intensive care unit (ICU). Communication is a critical component of PCC and patients and families have identified good communication as a critical aspect of high quality care in the ICU. Indeed, it is the primary mechanism that healthcare providers, patients, and families use to share information, convey the plan of care, discuss with the family and make decisions. Nurses provide the vast majority of bedside care and have the most opportunity to interact with patients and families. Nursing communication is thus vital not only between care givers but also between the nurse and the patient.

The following is a theoretical model for high quality patient centered communication as suggested by the American College of Critical Care Medicine with examples of behaviors and interactions and how these behaviors might contribute to specific outcomes.

According to this model (Fig. 1), patient-centered care has several definitions but encompasses five domains:

1. The biopsychosocial perspective with a focus on information exchange

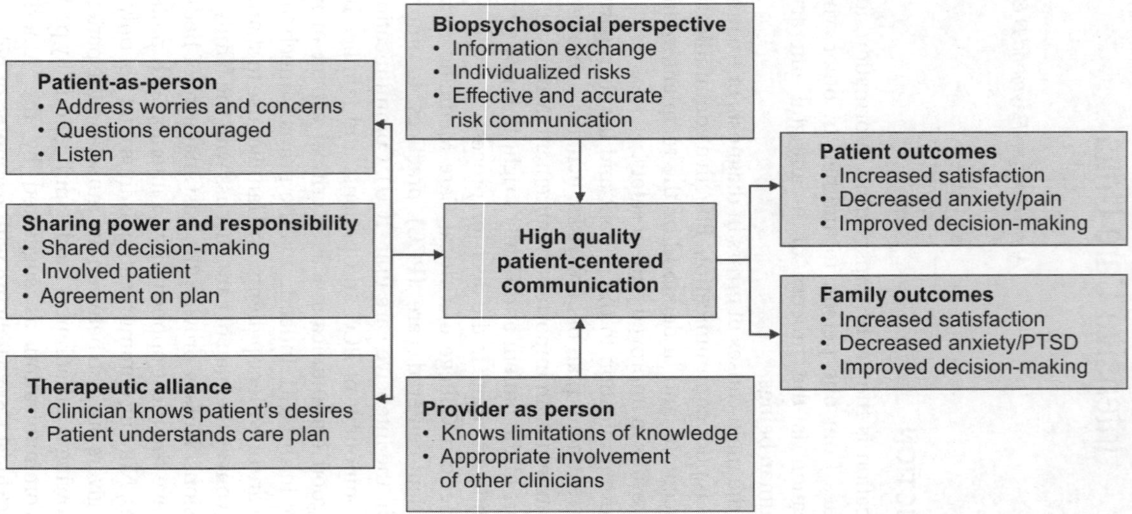

Fig. 1: Theoretical model for high quality patient centered communication as suggested by the American College of Critical Care Medicine

2. The "patient-as-person"
3. Sharing power and responsibility
4. The therapeutic alliance
5. The "clinician-as-person".

Patient-centered care and nurse communication has a large impact in the treatment of ICU patients. It has been observed that nurses usually communicate more on a personal level to patients and their families. They involve less in clinical discussions with patients or families since this responsibility is usually taken by the clinician which is the best thing to do since it involves technicalities. Also, it is advisable that since the clinician is more knowledgeable about the patient condition, he/she communicated to the patient/family regarding the same in order to avoid duplication or confusion regarding the same.

However, on a personal domain, nurses have many interactions with patients and families in the patient-as-person domain and several studies have emphasized the importance of this role. Families appreciate nurses who treat the patient and family as persons in addition to sharing personal details about themselves. Patients have reported that nurses are more friendly and less controlling than physicians, emphasizing the enhanced role nurses play in the patient-as-person domain of PCC.

Patient-centered critical care requires a collaborative approach that takes advantage of all the skills and expertise provide by individual members of the ICU team. It is unrealistic to expect an individual provider to provide all aspects of patient-centered communication with each individual patient and family. Nurses provide the vast majority of bedside care to patients and families and accordingly have the most opportunities to communicate with them.

In the ICU setting where most patients are ventilated or sedated, verbal communication usually takes a back seat. Head nods, gestures, mouthing words, and, writing are more common modes of communication between the nurse and the patient. The use of alphabets or word communication boards or other forms of augmentative and assistive communication aids like picture books may be used. Gestures generated by the patients usually represent basic needs like pain, need to suction, thirst, sleep, etc. and are usually interpreted with ease within the context of the ICU. In some successful interactions, "mirroring," or nurses' replication of gestures initiated by patients to affirm their meaning, is a technique that is helpful for gestural communication by nonspeaking patients.

Barriers in Communication

For every patient or family member, barriers to effective communication need to be identified, if any. This must be done during the initial assessment itself. The following barriers may be discovered: language barrier, lack of interest, cognitive problems, anxiety, depression, etc. Barriers in communication may be external or internal (Table 1).

Table 1: Barriers in communication

External	*Internal*
• External sounds • Distance • Delivery of the speaker • Unfamiliar language	• Personal concerns • Prejudice and biases • Fatigue • Physical or cognitive disabilities • Uninteresting subject • Judgmental

It is important to identify the barrier and take steps accordingly to overcome these barriers for effective communication.

The following practices are advised in an ICU setting for nurse patient communication:

- Good history taking and knowing likes and dislikes of patient helps in communication.
- Always get attention of the patient.
- Speak out patient's name aloud or gently touch to get a response.
- Wait for the patient to acknowledge.
- Establish a clear YES/NO signals, for example, a thumbs up sign for Yes and thumbs down sign for No.
  Some patient can use gestures to communicate their needs.
- Keep printed gesture dictionary in the patient's room or bed side.
- Teach patient universal gestures.
- Picture books are also used as an easy way to communicate.
- Pain assessment is very important for which the Wong Baker faces may be used.
- Procedure boards may be used to explain procedures like tracheostomy, central line insertion, CT/MRI/X ray.

Since, the patient is completely under the care of the nurse in the ICU setting, communication between the nurse and the patient is a vital component of patient care. It is important that the nurse understands his/her patients' needs and is able to communicate effectively. The vulnerable condition of the patient who may be intubated or sedated or under restraints must be taken into account for this. Empathy plays a big role in this scenario. Even a comforting touch, a reassuring look goes a long way in ICU patient care.

COMMUNICATION BETWEEN NURSE AND OTHER CARE GIVERS

Effective communication between the care givers is also of paramount importance since gaps in this may lead to medical errors. Effective communication which is timely, accurate, complete, unambiguous, and understood by the recipient must be used to prevent errors and improve patient safety and quality of care. Communication may be written, electronic or verbal.

A standardized communication approach to hand over patient information is required under the following circumstances but is not limited to:

- Change of patients' care from one care provider to another including change of provider at the end of shift, for intra-procedural change, or change of assignment within a shift.
- Nurse-to-Nurse mid-shift reports related to new patient admissions or changes in patients' plan of care/status.
- Assuming temporary responsibility for care when staff leaving unit for a short period of time.
- Notification to providers for critical laboratory, and any other critical diagnostic test results, or a change in patient status as appropriate.
- Transferring a patient from one internal level of care to another, including to/from procedural areas and admissions from the emergency department.

Standardized checklists may be used at every point where transfer of care occurs between care givers or different units such as:

- Checklists
- Shift endorsement tool
- Tracer chart
- In house transfer form
- Consultation/Referral record.

ISBAR TOOL

The ISBAR (Identify, Situation, Background, Assessment and Recommendation) is a mnemonic created to improve safety in the transfer of critical information. It originates from SBAR, the most frequently used mnemonic in health and other high-risk environments such as the military. The "I" in ISBAR is to ensure that accurate identification of those participating in handover and of the patient is established.

Identification

- Identify yourself, name and location.
- Confirm identification of the person to whom you are speaking to.
- Patient name, unique hospital identification (UHID) number and age.

Situation

- Patient's chief complaint/history of presenting illness
- Pertinent Physicians involved related to current condition
- Diagnosis and admit date
- Describe what is going on with the patient.

Background

- Any current/pertinent medical history related to the condition, which may include, but is not limited to:
  - Past history
  - Allergies
  - Current medications/relationship to condition
  - Comorbidities affecting patient status
  - Cardiac status (*as applicable*), with telemetry monitoring information
- Pertinent procedures/tests completed
- Most recent vital signs, blood glucose, pertinent laboratories
- Vascular access device (VAD) information (access sites, fluids, drips, etc.)
- Oxygen liter flow-if applicable
- Hearing/visual/cognitive/language barriers/mentation
- Patient mobility/Risk for fall
- Isolation/Infection control precautions—if applicable
- Diet restrictions if any.

Assessment

- **Pertinent** assessment changes/Exceptions to plan of care.

For example: Change in respiratory status, diaphoretic, Change in level and/or location of pain, anticoagulation therapy with elevated INR

This is what I think is happening........

CRITICAL RESULT INTIMATION

Any result that reveals a condition that could be potentially life-threatening to the patient and/or merit immediate medical intervention is termed as critical result.

We need to provide a mechanism for notifying the ordering physician, other licensed health care providers and patient/patient representative with critical results for diagnostic and investigational test and to promote effective communication amongst healthcare professional, that is timely, accurate, and complete and understood by the recipient to reduce errors and improved patient safety.

Investigation and diagnostic setting includes, but not limited to:

- Clinical laboratory
- Imaging services
- In-patient clinical areas.

The patient's full name and unique hospital identification number must be used to identify the patient. ***(Always use at least two patient identifiers not including the patient's location/room number/bed number)***

Communicate the result to the/ordering physician/resident doctor emphasizing that the result is **critical**. Ensure that the complete verbal/telephone critical test result is written down, read back and confirmed by the receiver.

Read Back

The receiver should write down the result, read back to the sender the information that has been written. When the Resident doctor has been informed about the critical result he/she should perform immediate medical intervention to stabilize the patient and notify the requesting/ordering physician.

The test result should be confirmed by the individual who gave the critical result.

Confirm

The sender shall listen carefully while the information is being read back.

The sender shall confirm to the receiver whether the information read back are correct, if not the sender shall correct the information. The same protocol shall be followed when correcting the information.

If the sender did not confirm, the receiver shall ask the sender to confirm.

Documentation

The critical result intimation register shall be maintained in all diagnostic areas and point of care test locations. It must indicate all the necessary information in communicating critical results including:

- Number of failed attempts
- Actions taken when delay occurs
- When physician cannot be contacted.

All critical results reported verbally or through phone should be verified. The receiver should **write down** the complete test result and "**read back**" the result, the sender **confirms** the reported results. The reporter should document the same in the critical result intimation register.

Telephone/Verbal Orders

To ensure that the effective communication of telephone and verbal medication orders, other physician orders and clinical investigations results is timely, accurate, complete, unambiguous and understood by the recipient as this reduces errors and results in improved patient safety.

A "verbal order" is defined as a medication order given by duly authorized prescribers, when the physician is present and it is an emergency situation, as he or she is performing sterile procedure or involved in a life-saving intervention.

A "telephone order" is defined as a medication order given by duly authorized prescribers, when the physician is present and it is an emergency situation, as he or she is performing sterile procedure or involved in a life-saving intervention.

Telephone and verbal orders must not be accepted for controlled, narcotic and chemotherapy medications.

Verbal and telephonic orders, other than medication orders shall be given when it is in the best interest of the patient in a manner that avoids delay in patient care and treatment. All verbal and telephonic communications of medication orders and other physician orders should follow the verbal and telephonic communication protocol as follows:

- The receiver shall write down the information communicated verbally or by phone.
- The receiver shall read back the information written to the sender.
- The sender shall confirm that the information read back were accurate.
- The concerned doctor shall sign the order within 24 hours.

Exceptions to the verbal and telephonic communication protocol are when orders including medication orders are given during an emergency and life-saving procedures, "code blue" or during surgical procedures, however, repeating the order and confirmation are still required.

The sender of the telephone order needs to identify himself/herself, the patient and the receiver of the order. Telephone orders are immediately written in the patient record by the individual receiving the order.

It is a common practice by some to record all telephone orders by the registered nurse in the medication administration record using a telephone order sticker. The telephone order is read back verbatim to the prescriber for verification of accuracy. Repeating the order back to the prescriber without writing it first is not acceptable.

The readback applies to all telephone orders.

Telephone orders are reviewed and countersigned by the prescriber or another physician member of the team caring for the patient as soon as possible, but not later than 24 hours. This could be done in the "telephone order sticker" or in the Doctors' orders.

27

CHAPTER

Documentation in Intensive Care Unit

Judith Vasan, Vajrapu Rajendra

INTRODUCTION

Generally for the nurses patient care takes a priority over paperwork, hence most nurses feel discouraged and overwhelmed by the amount of mandatory documentation to be completed. A good knowledge of proper documentation benefits patients in particular and the attending multidisciplinary team in general.

As per Patricia Benner, a nursing theorist, "nursing is relational and cannot be adequately described by strategies that leave out content, context and function".

Nursing documentation should be well organized and complete and should help to communicate patient information in a comprehensive way to the multidisciplinary team, useful as an educational tool, garner accreditation, reimbursements and also protect the nurse as well as the institute in legal aspects.

In the following pages you would be able to gain knowledge on various aspects of documentation starting from its meaning, need and purpose, professional and legal aspects, precautions when using electronic documentation, various forms and formats, special situations including consents, incident reporting, patient's personal property documentation and 24 hours record checks, etc.

What is Nursing Documentation?

Documentation in nursing practice anything written or electronically generated that describes the status of the client while on the care or services given to that client (Perry A and Potter G, 2010). Patients/client record gives information about the care given and the response to that care.

Examples of documents includes admission registers, referral forms, Kardexes, treatment sheets, mortality records, observation charts, ward round records, shift notes and anecdotal notes, etc. (American Association of Nurses, 2005).

Documentation also acts as a formal legal document that gives details of a client's management. Throughout the world, it is well accepted that "*if not documented, then it was not done, thus documentation should be complete and accurate* (Wetter, 2005)", documentation is not optional.

HISTORICAL PERSPECTIVES

Since the time of Florence Nightingale, nurses have viewed documentation as a very important aspect of their professional practice. Nightingale described the need to document proper use of air, light, warmth, cleanliness and proper selection of diet with an aim of collecting and retrieving data to aid in proper patient management.

Virginia Henderson, a nurse theorist, promoted the use of documentation in the nursing care plans to communicate during the 1930's. However, the nursing documentation was discarded after the patient had been discharged. Since 1970's nursing documentation has become more important reflecting the changes in nursing practice, regulatory agency requirements and legal guidelines. Nursing documentation has also evolved as an important mechanism in determining monetary reimbursement of the care provided to clients/patients (Iyer et al. 2006).

Documentation also stands in as a source of evidence of each health care provider's accountability in the delivery of care, therefore, professional nurses are expected to document the care given to patient/client in all settings (Crisp, Potter, Taylor and Perry, 2005; American Nurses Association, 2005).

Patient/client's record gives a lot of information about the care given and the response to that care. Examples of the documents used by health care providers are admission registers, referrals forms, Kardexes, treatment sheets, mortality records, images (X-rays, ultrasound scans, and magnetic resonance imaging), observation charts, ward round records, supervisors report, shift management reports and clinical anecdotal notes, etc. (American Association of Nurses, 2005).

PRINCIPLES OF DOCUMENTATION

Written communication should follow the guidelines of good communication and should be simple, clear, pertinent and above all, it should be accurate. Every nurse/health care professional must be familiar with their organizational policies or procedures related to documentation so as to operate within what is acceptable and avoid getting into problems. The following are general principles that should be observed as regards documentation (American Nurses Association, 2005).

Be Objective

Documentation on what is seen and heard should be made and not conclusions. A few examples of events documented could be during an assessment, when one observes a client having some bleeding he/she should indicate how much blood has been lost/or is being lost, whether it is clear, gushing, oozing and the source of the bleeding. After a nursing intervention, one should identify the patient's reaction, e.g. after giving medications, one should record the patient's response as well as time, dosage, route and description of any side effects.

If it is collection of a specimen, one should indicate the time it was obtained, the characteristics and where applicable where the specimen was taken and received. If a patient declines to take his treatment or any procedure, it is good to ensure that it is as well documented.

Be Specific

Ambiguous statements and generalization in documentations should be avoided. It is common practice when handing over reports to hear statements such as "the patient had a fair night" or "the patient had an uncomfortable night", these do not give any specific information. If the nurse instead records that the patient was up 10 times because of diarrhea during the night, this would tell why that particular patient had an uncomfortable night.

When documenting what the patient said verbally, the health care provider should use direct quotes. One should not document what someone else said about the patient. If there was an emergency that one had to attend to and did not document immediately, then is should be done as soon as possible as a "late entry" stating when the action was done and when it was entered.

Be Clear and Consistent

It is important to make sure that all hospital records are written in proper sentence structure, spelling and neatly written. Standard abbreviations should be used, one should not invent his/her own because this may bring about confusion and misinterpretations. It is paramount to append signatures date and time for all procedures done on the patient.

Record All Relevant Information Including Communications with Other Members of the Health Team

A scenario that illustrates this is when for instance, a new patient arrives in the ward at 10.00 PM in the night and the doctor on duty was called at 10.30 PM to see the patient and he/she did not turn up. A repeat call was made at 11.30 PM and the doctor said "I will be coming soon", all of this conversation by phone should be documented stating the times, names and the responses obtained. One should also document all the other procedures that were being done while waiting for the doctor to come. Under many circumstances, disputes erupt when doctors deny being called or notified especially whenever a legal issue arises.

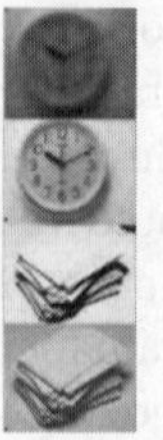

Guidelines for documentation
- Factual basis
- Accuracy
- Completeness
- Currentness
- Organization
- Confidentiality
- Pertinent data

Fig. 1: Guidelines for documentation

Respect Confidentiality

Patient records should only be shared with the health care team participating in the management of that particular patient and not with any one else. It is unethical to discuss patients' care/management over "tea or coffee time" as this amount to breach of confidentiality which is illegal.

Recording Errors

Whenever an error is made during documentation, whitener should not be used on the patient's chart, this is illegal and may be considered as a cover-up. This should be crossed out in a single line and an "error" written on it followed by a signature and the correct statement written (Clinical Audit and Nursing Research, MTRH, 2011).

PURPOSES OF DOCUMENTATION

Documentation serves three purposes:
1. It facilitates communication
2. It promotes safe and appropriate nursing care and
3. It meets professional and legal standards.

Communication

Through documentation, nurses communicate to other health care providers their nursing assessment, diagnosis of a client's condition, the plan of care, interventions and the outcomes of the interventions.

Safe and Appropriate Nursing Care

When nurses document the care they provide, other members of the health care team are able to review the documentation and plan their own contributions to safe and appropriate care. Documentation also provides data for research and workload management, both of which have the potential to improve health outcomes.

Professional and Legal Standards

Documentation is a comprehensive record of care provided to a client. It demonstrates how a nurse has applied nursing knowledge, skills and judgment (CRNBC Standards of Practice).

Documentation is generally accepted as evidence in legal proceedings. It establishes the facts and circumstances related to the care given and assists nurses to recall details about a specific situation. A practice environment that has the necessary systems, supports and policies in place to enable nurses to document appropriately is fundamental to safe client care.

Vigilance is required to ensure high standards in record-keeping, whether records are in written or electronic form. The audit of patient documentation is a facet of risk management, and can help to promote quality (NMC, 2002) as it means standards can be assessed and areas for improvement identified (Dimond, 1999).

DOCUMENTATION IN CRITICAL CARE SETTINGS

As with any specialty area critical care has its own documentation standards based on patient's condition, technology used and internal standards. As patients in critical care require more frequent documentation the ICU flow sheets are designed in such a way that documentation could be simplified.

The first encounter with the patient in critical care involves the documentation of the ICU nursing assessment which involves the patients details, health history, physical examination, medications, allergies, drugs and other substance abuse, pain, activities of daily living and family support systems, advance directives if any.

Documentation of periarrest conditions presents a challenge to the nurse. The nurse must anticipate and recognize deteriorating conditions and document specific details in rapid succession in an extremely stressful situation. To accomplish this task, a code sheet may be used during arrest and resuscitation. The code sheet, progress notes, monitor strips, and flow sheet must demonstrate consistent recording of timed events to accurately reflect the care provided.

In ICUs, it is not uncommon for numerous physicians to be involved in a patient's care. The nurse must coordinate and organize the implementation of prescribed treatments and ensure that information is communicated to the appropriate physicians (AACN, 2008). A nurse's failure to notify a physician can be an act of omission resulting in liability (Wacker Guido, 2014).

Different Types of Charting

- Narrative charting
- Charting by exception
- Problem oriented charting
- Focus charting.

The next is the flow sheet gives clinical data such as vital signs, assessments, intake/output, arterial blood gas (ABG), hemodynamic monitoring, medication administration, intracranial pressure monitoring, cuff pressure readings, ventilator

Adult Nursing Assessment Form

GLOBAL HOSPITALS

Patient label	Unit/Consultant:

Admission profile

Date admitted: Time admitted: Patient arrival: Walking/Wheelchair/Stretcher

Patient accompanied on Admission: Yes/No If Yes, Name: ____ Relation: ____

Contact person (Name): ____ Relation: ____ Phone No: ____

Languages known: ____ Interpreter required: Yes/No

Educational status: Primary/Higher Secondary/Graduate/Post Graduate

Admitted from ☐ A and E ☐ OPD ____

Source of information: ☐ Patient ☐ Family ☐ Caregiver ☐ Other ____

Presenting complaints: ____ Onset ____

Health history (with duration)

☐ Cancer:	☐ HTN:	☐ Hepatitis:	☐ Renal:
☐ Respiratory:	☐ Diabetes:	☐ Stroke:	☐ Musculoskeletal:
☐ Cardiac:	☐ GI:	☐ Seizures:	☐ Mental health:
	☐ Hematology	☐ Glaucoma:	☐ Others:

Surgical history: ____

Known allergies/Adverse reactions:

Known or suspected allergies to :		Name of allergen/drug and description of reaction
1. Medication:	Y/N	
2. Blood transfusion:	Y/N	
3. Food:	Y/N	
4. Others:	Y/N	

Fig. 2: Nursing initial assessment form—ICU

settings, laboratory data and other ancillary departmental information. The flow sheets provide an ongoing, continuous monitoring over time.

Next to the nursing initial assessment and the flow sheets you could also use the narrative notes in the nurse's progress notes. The progress notes is devised to record patient status and track changes in condition. The progress notes gives the patients problems and needs, pertinent nursing observations, nursing reassessments, interventions and patients response to the interventions and progress towards meeting expected outcomes (Lippincott Williams and Wilkins, 2008).

Nursing care plans which include patient data, allergies, medication to be administered, treatment to be carried out, diagnostic investigations, IV therapy and other measures, nursing diagnosis, plan and interventions to be carried out, implementation and evaluation, end-of-life care orders, consultations to be informed, permitted activities and functional limitations, assistance needed and safety precautions if needed (Banet GA, et al. 2006).

GHG/AGHLBN/NUR/019

Clinical chart

Patient label

AWARE GLOBAL HOSPITALS more to life

DOA: Height (cm): BMI:

																										Pains score
Date																										
Postoperative day																										
Hospital day																										
Temperature		AM			PM			AM			PM			AM			PM			AM			PM			
C	F	2	6	10	2	6	10	2	6	10	2	6	10	2	6	10	2	6	10	2	6	10	2	6	10	
41.1°	106°																									10
40.5°	105°																									9
40°	104°																									8
39.4°	103°																									7
38.8°	102°																									6
38.3°	101°																									5
37.7°	100°																									4
37.2°	99°																									3
36.6°	98°																									2
36.1°	97°																									1
35.5°	96°																									0
Pulse rate (min)																										
Respiration (min)																										
Blood pressure (mm of Hg)																										
SPO_2 (If required)																										
Weight (Kg)																										
Type of diet																										
Bowel movement																										
Antibiotic day																										
Total intake (mL)																										
Total output (mL)																										
Well's score																										
Mews score																										
Fall risk reassessment score																										
Signature/Emp. ID																										
Signature of UI/Sup.																										

Contd...

Contd...

Diagnosis and prognosis/Surgery done	Apache	LIS/SOFA	Wong baker face scale
Drug allergies	SAPS II	NIHSS	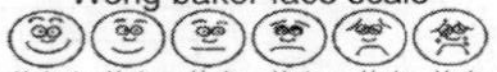

100	200	300	400	500	600	700			
							Investigation		
							HB/PCV		
							TLC		
							PLEM		
							ESR		
							Platelets		
							Smear TG/BF		
							Urea		
							Creatinine		
							NA/K/CL		
							PT/INR/APTT		
							D Dimer		
							Lactate		
							PCT		
							BT/CT		
							BIL D/I		
							SGPT/SGOT		
							ALKP		
							GGPT		
							Sprotein		
							ALB/GLO		
							Amyl/Lipase		
							CPK		
							LDH		
							TROP T/I		
							BNP		
							Dengue		
							Lepto		
							MP PV/PF		

Fluid bal	I/O				
Size	No of Day	No of time changed previous site	Fixed at	Cumulative Balance	
ETT/TP				Min BP	
Suction C/O				Max BP	
CVC/PL				Min Temp	
Art line				Max Temp	
PA/IABP				Min GRBS	
Foleys				Max GRBS	
Vent tube				Min PR	
HME/Heated				Max PR	
HD sheath				Min RR	
TPI				Max RR	
RT				Sleep quality	
MODE std by/pacing		Regular/missing (pacing)			
	No. units	Bag Nos.			
FFP					
PRBC/WH BL					
RDP/SDP					
Cryoppt					
Others					
Events					
C/S	Date	Report			
Urine					
Blood					
ET SEC/sput					

Fig. 3: Intensive care unit flowchart

GHG/AGH/IPR/-005

AWARE GLOBAL HOSPITALS more to life

Progress Sheet

Patient name: ....
IP No:............................ Age/Sex ....

Date and time	Clinical notes	Physician's order	Signature with name
Any change in care plan:			
Information patients/Attendants:			

Page No...................

Fig. 4: Nursing progress notes

All patients admitted to the ICU must have prophylactic strategies implemented in accordance with practice guidelines to prevent or decrease the incidence of complications like deep vein thrombosis, skin breakdown, VAP, CRBSI and infection control, etc. (Gerard J Criner, Rodger E Barnette, Gilbert E D'Alonzo, 2005).

Documentation of Restraints Use

Documentation includes who orders the restraints and the reason for restraints including the type of restraints use and the assessments following restraint use. In particular documentation has to describe less restrictive interventions before the use of physical or chemical restraints (Guido, 2010).

Care Bundle Checklist

Care bundle checklists helps in completeness of bundle care to prevent common mishaps in the care of critically sick patients.

Nursing Care Documentation

Date: _/_/_
Document code:

(Morning shift: 8 am – 2 pm/Evening shift: 2 pm–8 pm/Night shift 8 pm–8 am)

Patient label Name: ________ Age: ______ Sex: Male/Female IP No:	Hospital day: ICU day POD:		Diagnosis: Current/Potential problem:
Be fast: Mews/Pews:	Vip score:	DVT Score:	Braden score: Fall risk score:

Lines and tubes with days →	PL: LT/RT	EJV: LT/RT	CVC: LT/RT	ART L: LT/RT	Dalysis: LT/RT	Foley's:	ICD: LT/RT	ET/TT:	Others:

Nurshing care plan

I	Nurse applies nursing theory of king goal Attainment for mutual goal setting to plan Nurse patient contact hours at the beginning of each shift_hrs	II. Nursing care plan (care inclusion and modifications) after doctors rounds/Clinical rounds: 1. 2. 3. 4. 5.	Referrals: 1. 2. 3.

III Charting by PIE–Problem implementation evaluation

	Need/problem	Plan	Nursing care implementation	Evaluation	Reassessment	RN sign/ Emp no
	Identification based on assessment	Self-care deficit identified	Care implemented	Modified care planned and implemented	Patient response/ RNs observation/ instruction for care continuity	
1.	Hygiene and comfort need					
2.	Rest and sleep					
3.	Safety:1, Prevention of infection, injury, fall and complication 2. Care of tubes, drains and testraints/devices 3. Tissue viability management 4. Providing therapeutic environment					
4.	Activity: Exercise/positioning/ safe mobilization/					
	Transportation/ ambulation/ rehabilitation					
5.	Airway, breathing, oxygenation and perfusion					
6.	Nutritional need (Normal, Modified or therapeutic)					
7.	Elimination need—bowel and bladder					
8.	Fluid and electrolyte need					
9.	Physiologic response—MEWS/PEWS/Vital signs/ cardinal signs					
10.	Sensory needs, Expression, Feeling and reaction communication;					
11.	Psychosocial and spiritual needs (Non-pharmacological)					
12.	Age and disease specific physical, emotional and developmental needs					
13.	Health education and preparation for discharge involving family/information counseling and guidance					
14.	Advanced/special care like VAC dressing/burns dressing/ ostomy care/bipap care/end of life care etc.					

Chart by exception

Sl No.	Time		For information	Continue care
1.				
2.				
3.				
4.				
5.				
6.				
7.				
8.				

Pending	Referral consultation;	Procedures: Primary consultant visit: Used ward stock replaced: Yes/No/NA	Reports-Lab Reports-Radiology Med from pharmacy:
	Crash trolley items replaced: Yes/No/NA		
Handed over by— Name:		Taken over by—Name:	
Sign and ID No:		Time: Sign and ID No:	
Team leader/Nurse incharge/Supervisor—Name:		Sign and ID No:	

Fig. 5: Nursing care plans in intensive care unit

GHG/AGH LBN/CLIN/45

AWARE GLOBAL HOSPITALS more to life

DVT/PE Risk Factor Checklist—FORM A

Patient label

No.	Risk factors	Yes/No
1.	Age >40 years	
2.	Prior history of DVT/PE	
3.	Family H/o thrombosis	
4.	Hypercoagulable state (inherited or accquired)	
5.	Non hemorrhagic stroke <1month	
6.	Spinal cord injury	
7.	Diabetes mellitus	
8.	Systemic arterial hypertension	
9.	Myocardial infarction	
10.	Hospitalization with medical illness such as pneumonia or CCF; stay in medical or surgical intensive care unit	
11.	Burns	
12.	Sepsis/severe infection	
13.	Trauma	
14.	Immobilizing >72 hours	
15.	Immobilizing lower extremity cast/traction	
16.	Cancer	
17.	Cancer therapy (hormonal chemotherapy or radiotherapy)	
18.	Pregnancy/postpartum period	
19.	Use of oral contraceptive containing estrogen	
20.	Obesity (BMI >30)	
21.	H/o immediate past long haul air travel	
22.	Major surgery	
23.	Cigarette smoking	
24.	Varicose vein	
25.	Indwelling central venous catheter, pacemakers and internal cardiac defibrilators	
	Staff signature:	
	Supervisor sign:	

Fig. 6: DVT assessment chart

Well's criteria for DVT risk assessment form - B

Assign a score of 1 if (YES) in parameter 1 to 9 and assign a score of -2 if (YES) in parameter no, 10

Sl No.	Parameters										
1.	Active cancer (on-going treatment or diagnosed within 6 months or palliative care)										
2.	Bedridden recently > 3 days or major surgery within four weeks										
3.	Calf swelling 3 cm compared with asymptomatic side, measured at 10 cm below tibial tubercle (Assess for both legs)										
4.	Collateral (non-varicose) superficial veins present (assess for both legs)										
5.	Entire leg swollen (assess for both legs)										
6.	Localized tenderness along the deep venous system (assess for both legs)										
7.	Pitting edema, greater in the symptomatic leg (assess for both legs)										
8.	Paralysis, paresis, or recent plaster immobilization of the lower extremity (assess for both legs)										
9.	Previously documented DVT (assess for both legs)										
10.	Alternative diagnosis to DVT as likely or more likely (Assess for both legs)/Comorbidity like ESLD/renal disease, renal failure, CCFcellulitis (commonly mistaken as DVT), dependent (stasis) edema, lymphatic obstruction, septic arthritis, cirrhosis, nephrotic syndrome, calf muscle tear or strain, Hematoma (collection of blood) in the muscle, sprain or rupture of a leg tendon, fracture.										
	Final scoring										
	DVT prophylaxis started Y/N										
	Nurse sign:										
	Name of the doctor informed:										
	Risk score interpretation (probablity of DVT)										
I	If score is > 2 then it's a high-risk patient, require clinical judgment for confirming diagnosis and treatment plan										
II	If score is between 1 to 2, then moderate risk patient, require clinical judgment for further radiology examination										
III	If score is <1 then low-risk patient, ensure no additional risk factors and age > 40 years, decision based on clinical judgment										

Fig. 7: Deep vein thrombosis (DVT) assessment chart

Braden scale for predicting pressure sore risk GHG/AGH LBN/NUR/01

Individuals with a total score of 16 or less are considered at risk 15–16 = low-risk. 13–14 = moderate risk 12 or less = high-risk.	Undertake and document risk assessment within in G hours of admission or first home visit. Reassess it there is a change in individual's condition and repeat regularity according to local protocol

Patient's Name	Evaluator name			Date of assessment			
Sensory perception Ability to respond meaningfully to pressure-related discomfort	1. Completely limited unresponsive ideas not moan, flinch, or grasp to painful stimuli, due to diminished level to consciousness or sedation OR limited ability to feel pain over most of body	2. Very limited Responds only to painful stimuli-cannot communicate discomfort except by moaning or restlessness or has a sensory impairment which limits the ability to feel pain or discomfort over ½ of body	3. Slightly limited Responds to verbal commands. but cannot always communicate discomfort or the need to be turned or has some sensory impairment with limits ability to feel pain or discomfort in 1 or 2 extremities	4. No impairment Responds to verbal commands. Has no sensory deficit which would limit abillity to feel or voice pain or discomfort			
Moisture Degree to which skin is exposed to moisture	1. Constantly moist skin is kept moist almost constantly by perspiration, urine, etc. Dampness is detected every time patient is moved or turned	2. Very moist skin is often, but not always moist, linen must be changed at least once a shift	3. Occasionally Moist skin is occasionally moist, requiring an extra linen change approxirnately once a day	4. Rarely moist Skin is usually dry, linen only requires changing at routine intervals			
Activity Degree of physical activity	1 Bedfast confined to bed	2. Chatirfas Ability to walk severely limited or non-existent. Cannot bear own weight and/or must be assisted into chair or wheelchair	3. Walks occasionally Walks occasionally during day, but for very short distances, with or without assistance. spends majority of each shift in bed or chair	4. Walks frequently Wails outside room at least twice a day and inside room at least once every two hours during waking hours			
Mobility Ablity to change and control body position	1. Completely immobile Does not make even slight changes in body or extremity position without assistance.	2. Very limited makes occasional slight changes in body or extremity position but unable to make frequent or significant changes independently	3. Slightly limited makes frequent though slight changes in body or extremity position independently	4. No limitation Makes major and frequent changes in position without assistance			
Nutrition Usual food intake pattern	1. Very poor Never eats a complete meal. Rarely eats more than ½ of any food offered. Eats 2 servings or less of protein (meat or dairy products) per day. Takes fluids poorly. Does not take a liquid dietary supplement OR is NPO and/or maintained on clear liquids or IV's for more than 5 days	2. Probably inadequate Rarely eats a complete meal and generally eats only about ½ of any food offered. Protein intake includes only 3 servings of meal or dairy products per day. Occasionally will take a dietary supplement or receives less than optimum amount of liquid diet or tube feeding	3. Adequate Eats over half of most meals Eats a total of 4 servings of protein (meat, dairy products) per day. Occasionally will refuse a meal, but will usually take a supplement when offered OR is on a tube feeding or TPN regimen which probably meets most of nutritional needs	4. Excellent Eats most of every meal. Never refuses a meal. Usually eats a total of 4 or more servings of meat and dairy products. Occasionally eats between meals. Does not require supplementation			
Friction and shear	1. Problem Requires moderate to maximum assistance in moving. Complete lifting without sliding against sheets is impossible. Frequently slides down in bed or chair, requiring frequent repositioning with maximum assistance. Spasticity, contractures or agitation leads to almost constant friction	2. Potential problem Moves feebly or requires minimum assistance. During a move skin probably slides to some extent against sheets-chair-restraints; or other devices. Maintains relatively good position in chair or bed most of the time but occasionally slides down	3. No apparent problem Moves in bed and in chair independently and has sufficient muscle strength to lift up completely during move. Maintains good position in bed or chair				
				Total Score			

Fig. 8: Braden Scoring Form

SPECIAL DOCUMENTATION PRACTICES

Cardiopulmonary Resuscitation Documentation

Documentation should include any observations prior to the code the time of initial call for help from the first responder and all assessments and interventions including advance directives. It should also include physicians name, time, any specifics regarding the patient's condition including essential data. When the patient is successfully resuscitated the time of return of spontaneous circulation and post-CPR therapeutic hypothermia status also to be documented.

Incident or Occurrence Reports

Incident reports are sometimes referred to as accident reports, critical incident reports, variance reports, or occurrence

AWARE GLOBAL HOSPITALS more to life

Special Consents

Informed consent for use of restrant

Section-1 (To be handed over to the patient/relatives)

(Please read this sheet before you consent for your treatment)

What is restraint?

"Restraint" means any method or device used to involuntarily limit freedom of movement, including, but not limited to bodily physical force, mechanical devices, or chemicals "Restraint" includes a chemical restraint, a physical restraint.

What are the types of restraints used GHHC?

- Physical : Bandages
- Pharmacological : Mild sedation
- Boxers
- Restraint in the form of cloth

Why my patient should be under restraints?

- It prevents injury form all
- Prevention of injury to self/other
- Provision of necessary treatment

What are the risks associated with restraining the patient?

- Loss of muscle tone
- Decreased mobility
- Frustration
- Constipation due to use of certain drugs. This is temporary.

Note : The above stated risks and complications are only illustrative in nature

The restrained individual will be under regular observation, and will have adequate opportunities for movement and toileting. A plan will be in place for eventually phasing out the use of restraints completely -or at least finding the least restrictive form of care that will meet the needs of that particular individual

The staff will monitor the patient for common side effects of restraint use, such as increasing weakness, other physical effects, fear, agitation and depression, staff will be prepared to address these problems if they occur.

Any other risks rarticular to the individual patient (To be filled by treating doctor/deputed by him)

....

....

....

Fig. 9: Restraint assessment form

reports. Incident reports are used to document an actual or potential accident or unexpected event.

Incidents may lead to litigation, and a nurse may be named in the 'lawsuit.' Nurses can minimize exposure to malpractice 'lawsuits' by paying careful attention to interpersonal relationships, using good communication techniques, and practicing as would any prudent nurse in a similar situation. It is important for nurses to understand and uphold institutional, professional, and legal standards of practice and work within their scope of practice. Improved patient outcomes and protection of nurses against 'lawsuits' occur with attention to detail.

Nurses can minimize the risk of litigation by providing safe, high-quality nursing care. Identifying potential problem areas, identifying risk areas in individual practice, and taking measures to minimize exposure to those risks may help nurses avoid malpractice claims.

The 10 most common allegations in nursing malpractice cases are as follows:

1. Patient falls
2. Failure to monitor

Special consents

Section - 2

Declaration by the patient

Recommended restrant: ....

Purpose for recommended restraint: ....

Recommended time for the use of restraint: ....

I, the undersigned acknowledge that Dr...........................has explained to me that the patient has to be restrained part of the treatment procedure.

I certify and acknowledge that I have read this complete form both section-1 and section-2 and same has been explained to me in a laguage understood by me. I nave been made aware about the pertinent and unexpected risks and complications that might be caused.

Any other Risks particular to the individual patient (To be filled by treating doctor/deputed by him)

....

....

....

I also understand that I have the right to refuse the use of restraint after understanding the potential benefits, purpose and risks associated with the treatment plan of my patient.

☐ I hereby give my consent to restrain my patient.
☐ I hereby 'Do Not' give the consent to restrain my patient.

Name of the/Guardian :............ Signature

Relation with the patient:................. Name of the patient/IP No.................

Name of the doctor taking consent:................. Signature ....

Witness Name :............................. Address ....

Date and Time:...............................

Additional remarks (If Any):...............................

Fig. 10: Restraint assessment form

3. Failure to ensure patient safety
4. Improper delivery of treatment
5. Failure to respond to patient needs
6. Medication error
7. Wrong dosage administered
8. Failure to follow hospital procedure
9. Improper technique
10. Failure to supervise treatment.
    (Wacker Guido, 2014)

When an incident occurs, the nurse should first assess the patient for the extent of any injury and provide measures to prevent further injury. If a patient sustains an injury, the nurse must take steps to protect the patient, himself or herself, and the employer. Most agencies maintain policies regarding incidents. It is important to follow these policies. Nurses should never assume negligence occurred when an incident occurs. Accidents can and do occur in the absence of negligence. The risk manager collects incident reports, summarize to detect patterns, root causes, trends and also to address the trouble spots.

GHG/AGH LBN/NUR/002

Fall Risk Assessment Form

AWARE GLOBAL HOSPITALS more to life

Patient Label

Risk factor	Yes	No	Score
1. History of failing: Has the patient had more than 2 fails in the last 6 months?	☐	☐	1
2. Medications: Is the patient taking 4 or more medication?	☐	☐	1
Does the patient take any out of the following types medications? ☐ Vasodilator ☐ Analgesics ☐ Laxatives ☐ Sedatives ☐ Antidepressants ☐ Antidepressants ☐ Anticonvulsants ☐ Diuretics ☐ Psychorogic ☐ Vestibular	☐	☐	1
3. Balance/Gait/Mobility: Does the patient suffer form any problem associated with balance?	☐	☐	1
Is the patient unsafe/unsteady when asked to stand up from a chair, or bed, walk 3 meters, turn and return to the chair/bed independently (immobil = no)	☐	☐	1
Does the patient require any assistive devices to walk? (immobile = no)	☐	☐	1
4. Sensory loss: Does the patient have uncorrected sensory deficits that limits functional ability?	☐	☐	1
☐ Vision ☐ Hearing ☐ Somatosensory (touch)	☐ ☐ ☐	☐ ☐ ☐	1 1 1
5. Communication : Have any language or communication barriers been identified, e.g. an inability to ask for help, or language not understood by all staff?	☐	☐	1
6. Continence and bowel problems/elimination: if any of the factors are checked the patient score is 1 ☐ The patient is incontient ☐ Toileting as independent ☐ Requires diapers ☐ The patient requires frequent toileting and prompting to toiled ☐ Needs assistance with toilet ☐ The patient requires noctumal toileting	☐	☐	1
7. Mental State: Is the patient experiencing: ☐ Arodety ☐ Depression ☐ Confusion ☐ Disorientation ☐ Wandering ☐ Decreased cooperation, insight, or judgement, especially regarding mobility Development delayed	☐	☐	1
8. Nutrition: Has the patient's food intake decreased in the past 3 months due to loss of appetite, digestive problems or chewing or swallowing difficulties"	☐	☐	1
Has the patient bed recent unintentional weight gain or loss in the last 3 months?	☐	☐	1
9. Acute illness: Does the patient's have any signs of acute illness, e.g. altred behaviour, pain, malaise, fever, urinary symptoms, or intrapartum or postpartum blood loss?	☐	☐	1
10. Functional behavior : Is the patient afraid that going about his daily routine puts him at a high risk (e.g. bathing, toileting)	☐	☐	1
7. Mental state: Is the patient experiencing: ☐ Arthritis ☐ Stroke/transient ischemic attack ☐ Cardiac condition ☐ Diabetes ☐ Parkinson's disease ☐ Peripheral nouropathy ☐ Dementia ☐ Respiratory ☐ Lower limb amputation ☐ Other neurological conditions ☐ Vestibutar disorder (e.g.: dizziness meniere's disease)	☐	☐	1
12. Mechanical or environmental restraints: Are any of the following devices being used? ☐ Intravenous therapy ☐ Drain Specity tupe ——— ☐ Foley's catheter ☐ Wrist or vest restraints	☐	☐	1
13. Surgery: Does the patient have any of the following medical conditions that his balance and mobility? if any of the above risk factore checked the patient score? ☐ Intraoperative blood loss more than 700ml. (non replaced) ☐ Postoperative confusion ☐ Hypertension ☐ Post operative confusion ☐ Postoperative blood loss more than 100 ml ☐ Neurological ☐ Hypothermia ☐ Nausea and vomiting ☐ Hypotension ☐ Tachycardia ☐ Hypotension ☐ Received blood products intraoperatively ☐ Urgency associated with bladder or bowel elimination	☐	☐	1
Results			
If the total score 1 - 2 Initiate fall pravention protocol I If the total score 3 - 9 Initiate fall prevantion protocol II If the total score 3 - 9 Initiate fall prevantion protocol III Please complete the revarse side of the page, which detalis each fall previous protocol			

Contd...

Consent

A patient or his/her legal representative's signed consent form is necessary for admission to the health care facility, invasive procedures, surgery and some treatment protocols (Guido, 2010). Special consents are needed for specialized procedures. When in cases there is refusal of treatment consents to refusal of treatment should be also documented. All consent forms to be completely filled, dated, timed and signed.

Death or Dying

Carefully document all events when you are caring for a dying patient. Document any advance directives, living wills, power of attorney or health care proxy who will be able to give consent when the patient is unable to do so. Document any special orders to be carried out in the care of a dying patient.

Organ and Tissue Donation

In the case of organ or tissue donation the clinical nursing documentation involves documentation of hemodynamic variables, electrolyte values, laboratory values, urine output,

Contd...

Full prevention protocol applicable to this patient ☐ Fall prevention protocol I ☐ Fall prevention protocol II ☐ Fall prevention protocol III	
Risk fall prevention protocol I	
Preventive measures	Tick when implemented
Orientate the patient to the surroundings	☐
Family, friends, or sitter to stay with patient, if needed, educate family or sister regarding fall prevention	☐
The patient bed is set at the lowest position possible	☐
The nursing call bell is secured with in easy reach Ambulatory assistive devices, if needed are kept within easy reach	☐
All ambulatory patients are encouraged to wear skid - proof footwear	☐
All staff members are responsible for eliminating environmental hazards,	☐
Teach the patients and patient's family to use non-mobile furniture for balance and support	☐
Atleast 2 side rails are locked in position while the patient is in bed, on a stretcher, or unattended.	☐
All wheels on beds and stretchers are kept in the locked position	☐
Staff alerted to make frequent visual checks	☐
Others	☐
Initiated By: Employee name ________ Signature ________ Employee number ________ Date ________ Signature of patient/Relative: ________	
Fall prevention protocol II (all to the measures in protocol I, in a addition to those listed below)	
Preventive measures	
The patient or family, or both, have been instructed to request help for any patient activity to the surroundings	☐
Family, friends, or sitter to stay with patient, if needed, educate family or sister regarding fall prevention	☐
All items used by the patients are with in easy reach of the patient	☐
Call bell within reach of patient to obtain assistance to mobilize	☐
A bowel and bladder routines is instituted, if applicable	☐
The patient has been reassessed for safe footwear the patient environment has been reassessed is well fit and clutter-free	☐
The use of assistive devices, if applicable, has been reinforced	☐
The patient has been reassessed for safe footwear	☐
A risk alert sign is displayed on the patient's door	☐
Staff alerated to make frequent visual checks	☐
Others	☐
Initiated By: Employee name ________ Signature ________ Employee number ________ Date ________ Signature of patient/Relative: ________	
Fall prevention protocol III (all of the measures in protocol I and II addition to those listed below)	
Preventive measures	
Frequently reorient and repetitively reinforce the patient's understanding of the call bell, and ensure it is with in easy reach.	☐
Family, friends, or sitter to stay with patient, if needed, educate family or sister regarding fall prevention	☐
Initiate the high fall risk identification, including positing a vulnerable patients sign on the door, and a notation in the patient health record,	☐
Consider the need for additional night lighting	☐
Increase observation of the patient as needed	☐
Consider a room assignment closer to the nursing station	☐
Assist the patient with all activities	☐
Notify the attending physician for a medication review, if applicable	☐
Evaluate the need for physical therapy, e.g., strengh training/alternatives and the use of assistive mobility devices	☐
A sister to remain with the patient 24 hours a day	☐
Stryker bed alarms are activated according to patient assessment	☐
Others:	
Initiated By: Employee name ________ Signature ________ Employee number ________ Date ________ Signature of patient/Relative: ________	

Fig. 11: Fall risk assessment form

apnea test, corneal and gag reflex, cold calorie test, Glasgow Coma Score, doll's eyes reflex, end of life care summary, family discussions, protocols and authorization permits should also be documented. Check if the consent forms for organ and tissue donation to the extent of completeness of documentation.

Patients Personal Property

Documentation of dental appliances, jewellery, personal mementos such as photographs, prostheses should also be made as per hospital policy in nurse's progress notes or separate forms. (Patricia A Potter, Anne Griffin Perry, Patricia, 2004).

Legal and Professional Risks in Documentation

When filling out your documentation consider that you protect your patient's interests as well as your own by completing documentation in a accurate and timely manner in accordance

SSI BUNDLE CHECK LIST

SSI BUNDLE CHECK LIST				D-1	D-2	D-3	D-4	D-5	D-6	D-7
Patient Name:	Age/Sex:		Control blood glucose levels							
Dept:	Uhid:	Ipno:	Hand hygiene							
Reason For Surgery	Doa		Dressing change							
Surgeon Name:	Time In:		Maintenance of normothermia							
No of persons in ot:										
Duration of surgery:		Time Out:								
Review date:		Sign:	**Signs and Symptoms**							
			Date							
Ssi bundle (At the time of insertion - Tick the following)			Fever (>38c)							
Hand washing (Surgical hand washing)			Erythema/Tenderness							
Maximal barrier precautions upon insertion (Cap, Mask, Gown, Gloves)			Purulent discharge							
Antiseptic solution for cleaning of the incision Area			Localized Swelling							
Sterile drape and asepsis maintained through out the procedure			Localized Pain							
Appropriate antimicrobial prophylaxis			Culture		Antibiotics					
Skin preparation										
Daily reviewed By										

CRBSI Bundle

CRBSI Bundle Check List										
Patient Name:		Age/Sex:	Port is flushed and free from blood clots							
Dept:	Uhid:	Ip No:	Line is well secured							
Reason for insertion		Doa:	Anchoring central line dated and time							
Inserted by Name:		Time:	Closed central line system							
Date of insertion:		Number of atteprnts:								
Date of removal:		Time								
Removed By:		Sign:	Signs and symptoms							
CRBSI Bundle (At the time of insertion – tick the following)			Date							
			Fever (>38c)							
Hand washing (surgical hand washing)			Redness							
Maximal barrier precautions upon insertion (cap, mask, gown, gloves)			Tenderness on insertion site							
Antiseptic solution for cleaning of the incision area			Pain							
Sterile drape and asepsis maintained through out the procedure			Pus discharge from insertion site							
Insert using aseptic technique			Culture		Antibiotics					
Review catheter necessity daily and remove prompty										
Daily reviewed by										

Fig. 12: Care bundle check list form

with standards of nursing care and failure to document leads to malpractice issues.

Professional organizations like American Nurses Association, Joint Commission on Accreditation of Health Care Organizations, centers for medicare and medicaid services have established that documentation should include the following:

- Ongoing assessments
- Variation from assessments
- Nursing care
- Patient status
- Relevant statements made by the patient
- Responses to therapy
- Medical treatment and patient teaching.

In order to ensure timely communication of the patients status document the current patients status and the time physician was contacted. (when unable to contact the physician, again document the next contact time and the response). Incase of errors or omissions label as "late entry" to state that it is out of sequence and also record the date and time the entry should have been made. Incase of corrections or alterations the corrections should be made immediately with the date and time along with the name/signature/employment number stating "error".

CAUTI Core Bundle

CAUTI Bundle Check List													
Cauti Bundle Check List		Sterile continuous closed drainage system	D-1	D-2	D-3	D-4	D-5	D-6	D-7				
Patient Name:	Age /Sex:	Proprty placed catheter											
Dept: Uhid:	Ip no:	Secured catheter											
Reason for insertion:		Empty box											
Inserted by Name:	Time	Meatal care											
Date of insertion:	Number of attepmts:												
Reason for insertion:													
Date of removal:	Time												
Removed By	Sign:	Signs and symptoms											
		Date											
Cauti bundle (At the time of insertion tick the following)		Fever (>38c)											
Hand washing surgical hand washing)		Dysuria											
Maximal barrier precautions upon insertion (Cap, mask, gown, gloves)		Suprapubic tenderness											
Antiseptic solution for cleaning the urethral meatus		Pain											
Sterile lubricant jelley (single use)		Costovertebral angle pain/ tenderness)											
Insert using aseptic technique		Culture	Antibiotics										
Review catheter necessity daily and remove prompty													
Daily reviewed by													

Ventilator Bundle Checklist

Signs and symptoms: Temp, TLC, purulent secretion, X-RAY new changes, more suction requirement culture report:

Date	Bed/ patient initials	ICU day	Sedative interruption/ Assessment for ready to extubation	Pud prophylaxis	Dvt. prophylaxis	Head end elevation 30°	Oral pool ±	Cuff leak ±	Cuff pressure checking yes/no	Ventilator tubing in position	Condensation/ blood in tubing filter nebulizer	Filter changed yes/no	Oral care/ hygiene

Fig. 13: Care bundle check list form

AWARE GLOBAL HOSPITALS more to life

Cardiopulmonary Resuscitation (CPR) Notes

Intake information/inital assessment

Patient name :		UHID no:		Age/sex:	
Date	Time of arrest	Location ☐ Prehospital ☐ Rooms	Type of arrest ☐ Cardiac ☐ Respiratory ☐ Cardiopulmonary	Code status ☐ Full ☐ DNR ☐ UNK	Weight (kg)

Initial ventilation via ☐ Mouth yo mouth / mask ☐ Ambu IV present ☐ Yes ☐ No	Condition of patient on code team arrival Unconscious ☐ Yes ☐ No; Breathing ☐ Yes ☐ No; Pulse present ☐ Yes ☐ No; cyanotic ☐ Yes ☐ No; Pupils dilated ☐ Yes ☐ No; Temparature ☐ Cold ☐ Warm

Intubated by	Time	Type	Size	COZ detector ☐ Yes ☐ No ☐ N/A	Breath sounds equal ☐ Yes ☐ No ☐ Repositioned	PCXR, post-intubation ☐ Yes ☐ No ☐ N/A
Peripheral IV start	Time	Site	Size	Solution	Central line ☐ Yes ☐ No ☐ N/A	

CPR continued throughout code as per ACLS guidelines

	Blood pressure	Pulse	Epinephrine	Vasopressin	Atropine	Lidocaine	Procainamide	Mgso4	Dopamine	Amiodarone	Noradrenalin	Sodium bicarbonate	Calcium gluconate	25% dextrose	Insulin						Defibrillation	Rhythm
Time	mm of Hg	Per min	mg	Units	mg	mg	mg	mg	cc/hr.	mg	mg	mg	mL	mg	Units						Joules	
Notes																						

Code outcome			Team members	
Time code stopped	Disposition following code ☐ Critical care ☐ Expired ☐ Other		Physician signature	
			RN	RN
Family notified ☐ Yes ☐ No	By		RN	RN
Patient notified ☐ None ☐ To coroner	☐ With patient (complete list) ☐ Given to family (complete list)		Respiratory	Respiratory
Corner notified ☐ N/A ☐ Yes ☐ No	Coroner name	Coroner number	Pharmacist	Pharmacist
Primary notified will sign death certificate ☐ Yes ☐ No ☐ Yes ☐ No ☐ N/A		Organ/tissue donation ☐ Yes ☐ No explaine	Scribe number	

Fig. 14: CPR form

Malpractice and Documentation

Legally it focuses on 4 elements:

1. Duty (obligation to provide care)
2. Breach of duty (failure to fulfill nursing obligation)
3. Causation (that the breach caused the injury)
4. Damage (the amount of money to be paid for the injury when proven): Lippincott Williams and Wilkins, 2009.

Confidentiality in Documentation

Nurses assume the primary role in maintaining confidentiality and in safeguarding the privacy of the medical records. Breaches in confidentiality can result from unintentional release of information, unauthorized entry into the patient's records or even any casual conversation that is overheard by others.

Liability in Documentation

1. Omission in critical thinking
2. Inadequate evaluation of patient's status
3. Missing or incomplete documentation of paient's condition

AWARE GLOBAL HOSPITALS
more to life

CODE BLUE/MEDICAL EMERGENCY NURSE'S NOTE		
DATE	TIME	

Fig. 15: CPR form

4. Missing documentation of communication of change in patient's condition to physician (Jones and Bartlett, 2011).

Computerized Nursing Documentation

The American Nurses Association and the American Medical Records Association offer guidelines in maintaining the confidentiality in maintaining computerized medical records:

- Never share your password or computer signature
- Be aware of your surroundings
- Logoff if not using your terminal
- Follow your hospital policy for correcting errors
- Make backup files.

IT and Nursing Documentation

Computer-based nursing documentation can have an enormous impact on the quality of nursing documentation. Aspects that may be improved are clarity, completeness and

AWARE GLOBAL HOSPITALS more to life

Evaluation of Code Blue

Purpose: To analyze the care provided in an arrest situation for adherence to established guidelines; to identify opportunities to improve performance; and to improve outcomes.

Location of code (check one)

☐ E.R | ☐ ICU | ☐ SICU | ☐ CTICU | ☐ MICU | ☐ O.T | ☐ Ward | ☐ Other: ______

Patient condition prior to the code (check all that apply)

☐ Unknown	☐ Abnormal lab results	☐ Post invasive procedure
☐ Unstable vital signs	☐ Medication problems	☐ Other ______

Code Critique ('any items identified as " some difficulties" or "not met" require action)	Std. met.	Std. met. some problems	Std. not met.	Comments
	Score 1	Score 2	Score 3	
Code Blue Activated/Announced according to policy				
BLS guidelines followed				
AE dapplied & apropriately utilized				
Airway established				
Nitil rhythm identified & documented				
Code team responded within 3 minutes				
Physician present within 5 minutes				
ACLS guidelines followed				
Defib pads/paddles placed properly and "clear" called before each shock				
IV present or established within 5 min.				
Equipment immediately available (list missing or needed items in comments)				
Equipment functioned properly (list issues in comments)				
Supplies immediately available (list missing or needed items in comments)				
Medications immediately available (list missing or needed items in comments)				
Primary nurse at bedside with patient record				
Code Blue record complete and signed by physician				
No complication of resuscitation (i.e. fractured ribs. pneumothorax. etc. Document in comments)				
Outcome of code	☐ Successful		☐ Unsuccessful	

Overall assessment of code

☐ Meet standards (all areas above must score1). No action necessary

☐ Opportunity for improvement identified. on adverse outcome all areas above must score either 1 or 2)*

☐ Standards not met (score of 3 in one or more areas). Refer for review and action plan

* Refer issues for resolution

Name of the Evaluator : Date :

Signature : Time :

Fig. 16: CPR form

the amount of documentation. Many studies confirm this. For example, Van Gennip et al. (1995), found in the evaluation of nursing documentation on three non-ICU wards in three hospitals that information was more complete, more readable and clearer. Kahl et al. (1991), reported more complete, timely, readable and correct documentation after the introduction of bedside terminals to a nursing documentation system on two wards. A detailed evaluation of completeness of documentation after introduction of a nursing information system with care planning was also performed by Larrabee (2001) in a 100-bed hospital. Within the first 6 months after the implantation, he did not find an improvement of completeness. However, after retraining of the users, the completeness of the documentation of both nursing assessment and intervention improved.

Another comprehensive evaluation was carried out by Newton (1995), who found, 3 months after the introduction of the computer-based care planning on 16 wards, an increase in completeness and quality of documentation, measured with a standardized instrument. For example, more patients now had an assessment or care plan, the problem list was more complete and more goals were evaluated than without the computer. A comparable increase in quality of documentation, as judged by the Joint Commission for Accreditation for Healthcare Organization (JCAHO) standards, was also found by Mcbride and Nagle (1996). Pabst et al. (1996), even found that nurses using a comprehensive nursing documentation system updated the care plans more often.

FURTHER READING

1. American Association of Critical-Care Nurses (AACN). AACN scope and standards of practice for acute and critical care nursing practice. Aliso Viejo, CA: American Association of Critical-Care Nurses; 2008.
2. American Nurses Association, House of Delegates. Implications of fatigue on patient safety and nurse safety. (Available from the American Nurses Association 8515 Georgia Avenue, Suite 400, Silver Spring; 2005.
3. American Nurses Association, Principles of documentation. Washington. DC. 2002.
4. Association of Perioperative Registered Nurses (AORN). Perioperative standards and recommended practices. Denver, CO: Association of Peri operative Registered Nurses; 2014.
5. Association of Women's Health, Obstetric and Neonatal Nurses (AWHONN). Standards for Professional Nursing Practice in the Care of Women and Newborns (7th ed.). Washington, DC: Association of Women's Health,Obstetric and Neonatal Nurses, 2009.
6. Banet, GA, et al. Effects of implementing computerized practitioner order entry and nursing documentation on nursing flow in an emergency department, Journal of Healthcare Information Management. 2000;20(2):45-54.
7. Complete guide to documenation 2nd Ed editors Linda Hager, Julie Menden Walters Kluwers/ Lippincott Williams & Wilkins 2008.
8. Complete Guide to Documentation 2nd (Edn), Linda Hager, Julie Menden Walters Kluwers, (Eds). Lippincott Williams and Wikins, 2008.
9. Crisp J, and Taylor C. (Eds). Potters and Perry's Fundamentals of Nursing, 2nd (Edn), Elsevier, Australia. 2005.
10. International Journal of Humanitites and Social Science. 2013; 3(6):238.
11. Kenner C, and Lott J. Comprehensive neonatal nursing: a physiological perspective. 5th edition. Philadelphia, PA: Saunders. 2013.
12. Lyer P, Camp N. Nursing Documentation: A Nursing Process Approach, originally published by St. (2005).
13. Mcbride S, Nagle L. Attitutes towards computers: a test of construct validity. Computers in Nursing. 1996;14:164-70.
14. Newton C. A study of nurses attitudes and quality of documents in computer care planning. Nursing standard. 1995;9:35-9.
15. Pabst MK, Scherubel JC, Minnick AF. The impact of computerized documentation on nurses use of time. Computers Nursing. 1996; 14(1):25-30.
16. Sullivan D. Guide to clinical documentation. Philadelphia, PA: F. A. Davis 2011.

17. The Joint Commission. 2014. Specifications manual for national hospital inpatient quality measures.http://www.jointcommission.org/specifications_manual_for_national_hospital_inpatient_quality_measures.aspx.
18. Wacker Guido, G. 2014. Legal and ethical issues in nursing. Upper Saddle River, NJ: Pearson Education.
19. Wetter D. The best defence is a good documentation offense, 2005.

28

CHAPTER

Defibrillation and Cardioversion

Vajrapu Rajendra, Judith Vasan

INTRODUCTION

Defibrillation is a process in which an electrical device called a defibrillator sends an electric shock to the heart to stop an arrhythmia resulting in the return of a productive heart rhythm.

Defibrillation is the definitive treatment for the life-threatening cardiac arrhythmias such as ventricular fibrillation and pulseless ventricular tachycardia.

Cardioversion is a synchronized administration of shock during the R waves or QRS complex of a cardiac cycle. It is administered usually in supraventricular arrhythmias.

During defibrillation and cardioversion, electrical current travels from the negative to the positive electrode passing through the myocardium. It causes all of the heart cells to depolarize simultaneously following, which sinus node resumes normal pacemaker activity.

Indications for defibrillation include the following:

- Pulseless ventricular tachycardia (VT)
- Ventricular fibrillation (VF)
- Cardiac arrest due to or resulting in VF.

Indications for electrical cardioversion include the following:

- Supraventricular tachycardia
- Atrial fibrillation
- Atrial flutter
- Ventricular tachycardia with pulse.

Defibrillation is an emergency maneuver and, when necessary, should be promptly performed in cardiac arrest scenario.

Cardioversion is almost always performed under sedation (short-acting agent such as midazolam). The only exceptions are if the patient is hemodynamically unstable or if cardiovascular collapse is imminent.

Equipment includes the following:

- Defibrillators, automated external defibrillators (AEDs), semi-automated—AEDs, standard defibrillators with monitors).
- Paddle or adhesive patch
- Conductive gel or paste

- ECG monitor with pulse oximeter
- Intubation kit
- Emergency pacing equipment
- Blood pressure cuff (automatic or manual)
- Intravenous access
- Suction device
- Crash cart with emergency medications.

PADDLE PLACEMENT

Paddle placement on the chest wall has two conventional positions: anterolateral and anteroposterior.

In the anterolateral position, a single paddle is placed on the left fourth or fifth intercostal space on the midaxillary line. The second paddle is placed just to the right of the sternal edge on the second or third intercostal space.

In the anteroposterior position, a single paddle is placed to the right of the sternum, as above, and the other paddle is placed between the tip of the left scapula and the spine. An anteroposterior electrode position is more effective than the anterolateral position for external cardioversion of persistent atrial fibrillation. The anteroposterior approach is also preferred in patients with implantable devices, to avoid shunting current to the implantable device and damaging its system.

Advanced cardiovascular life support (ACLS) measures should be instituted in preparing the patient, such as obtaining intravenous access and preparing airway management equipment, sedative drugs, and a monitoring device.

MONOPHASIC VERSUS BIPHASIC WAVEFORMS

Defibrillators can deliver energy in various waveforms that are broadly characterized as monophasic or biphasic.

Monophasic defibrillation delivers a charge in only one direction. Biphasic defibrillation delivers a charge in one direction for half of the shock and in the electrically opposite direction for the second half. Newer defibrillators deliver energy in biphasic waveforms. Biphasic waveform defibrillators deliver a more consistent magnitude of current. They tend to successfully terminate arrhythmias at lower energies than monophasic waveform defibrillators.

Energy Selection for Defibrillation or Cardioversion

In 2010, the American Heart Association issued guidelines for initial energy requirements for monophasic and biphasic waveforms.

Atrial fibrillation energy requirements are as follows:

- 200 Joules for monophasic devices
- 120–200 Joules for biphasic devices.

Atrial flutter energy requirements are as follows:

- 100 Joules for monophasic devices
- 50–100 Joules for biphasic devices.

Ventricular tachycardia with pulse energy requirements are as follows:

- 200 Joules for monophasic devices
- 100 Joules for biphasic devices.

Ventricular fibrillation or pulseless ventricular tachycardia energy requirements are as follows:

- 360 Joules for monomorphic devices
- 120–200 Joules for biphasic devices.

The most common complications are harmless arrhythmias, such as atrial, ventricular, and junctional premature beats.

Serious complications include ventricular fibrillation resulting from high amounts of electrical energy, digitalis toxicity, severe heart disease, or improper synchronization of the shock with the R wave.

Thromboembolization is associated with cardioversion in 1–3% of patients, especially in patients with atrial fibrillation who have not been anticoagulated prior to cardioversion. Current, the American College of Cardiology (ACC)/American Heart Association (AHA) guidelines recommend to anticoagulate for 3–4 weeks before and after cardioversion. The presence of an intracardiac thrombus should be excluded using transesophageal echocardiography prior to cardioversion if therapeutic anticoagulation has not been achieved.

Myocardial necrosis can result from high-energy shocks. Pulmonary edema is a rare complication of cardioversion. It is more common in atrial fibrillation due to valvular heart disease or left ventricular systolic dysfunction.

Painful skin burns can occur after cardioversion or defibrillation; they are moderate to severe in 20–25% of patients. They most likely are due to improper technique and electrode placement. It occurs less with use of biphasic waveform defibrillators and use of gel-based pads.

FURTHER READING

1. Link MS, Atkins DL, Passman RS, Halperin HR, Samson RA, White RD, et al. Part 6: electrical therapies: automated external defibrillators, defibrillation, cardioversion, and pacing: 2010 American Heart Association Guidelines for Cardiopulmonary Resuscitation and Emergency Cardiovascular Care. Circulation. 2010;122(Suppl 3):S706-19.

29

CHAPTER

Terminal Care of a Dying Patient

RK Mani

TERMINAL CARE IN DYING PATIENTS: PALLIATIVE CARE AND BEREAVEMENT

Death is an everyday occurrence in the critical care unit. For many, life-support interventions have not helped to mitigate their suffering, but have rather added the agony and burden of a prolonged dying process. Prolonged and futile life support has undoubtedly imposed enormous economic strain on patients and families. Potentially salvageable patients can be denied ICU care when scarce beds and resources are consumed in a futile search of cure where death appears inevitable. Setting goals appropriate to clinical situations of poor prognosis are an integral part of critical care. Quality critical care requires that the practice be well grounded in ethical principles and that the ICU staff are trained in the skills of end of life care. A consensus regarding the practices relating to EOL care in Indian ICUs should eventually lead to the evolution of appropriate legislation in keeping with the changing needs of critical care practice.

CHECKLIST FOR INITIATING END-OF-LIFE (EOL) DISCUSSIONS

1. Advanced age coupled with a poor premorbid state due to chronic debilitating diseases, e.g. advanced chronic obstructive pulmonary disease (COPD) requiring home oxygen and/or bilevel pressure support or with severe impairment of quality of life; advanced interstitial lung disease on oxygen therapy with failed medical treatment, chronic renal failure requiring long-term dialysis, chronic liver disease, advanced congestive heart failure.
2. Catastrophic illnesses with organ dysfunctions unresponsive to a reasonable period of aggressive treatment.
3. Prolonged coma (in the absence of brain death) due to acute nonreversible causes or chronic vegetative state.
4. Incurable chronic severe neurological states rendering meaningful life unlikely, e.g. progressive dementia, quadriplegia with ventilator dependency.

5. Progressive metastatic cancer where treatment has failed or patient refuses treatment.
6. Post-cardiorespiratory arrest, nonrestoration of comprehension after a few days.
7. Patient/family preference to limit life support or refusal to accept life support.

RECOMMENDATIONS

1. The physician has a duty to disclose to the capable patient or family, the patient's poor prognosis with honesty and clarity when further aggressive support appears nonbeneficial. The physician should initiate discussions on the treatment options available including the option of no specific treatment.
2. When the fully informed capable patient or family desires to consider palliative care, the physician should offer the available modalities of limiting life-prolonging interventions. The patient or family should be clearly made aware of the available options for the use of life-sustaining supports as follows:
   a. Full support
   b. Do not intubate (DNI) or DNR status
   c. Withholding of life support
   d. Withdrawal of life support
   e. Palliative care.

   Pending consensus decisions or in the event of conflicts between the physician's recommendations and the family's wishes, all existing supportive interventions should continue. The physician however, is not morally obliged to institute new therapies against his/her better clinical judgment.
3. The discussions leading up to the decision to withhold life-sustaining therapies should be clearly documented in the case records, to ensure transparency and to avoid future misunderstandings. Such documentation should mention the persons who participated in the decision-making process and the treatments withheld or withdrawn.
4. The overall responsibility for the decision rests with the attending physician/intensivist of the patient, who must ensure that all members of the caregiver team including the medical and nursing staff agree with and follow the same approach to the care of the patient.
5. If the capable patient or family consistently desires that life support be withdrawn, in situations in which the physician considers aggressive treatment nonbeneficial, the treating team is ethically bound to consider withdrawal within the limits of existing laws.
6. In the event of withdrawal or withholding of support, it is the physician's obligation to provide compassionate and

effective palliative care to the patient as well as attend to the emotional needs of the family.

7. Palliative care support includes adequate control of pain, respiratory distress, psychological stress and attention to symptoms such as nausea, vomiting or constipation. Spiritual rites and environment have an important role to play in the holistic care of the patient.

Bereavement is a universal human experience and potentially dangerous to health. It is associated with a high mortality, and up to a third of bereaved people develop a depressive illness. Post-bereavement support is therefore of vital importance. Help targeted at those most at risk has been shown to be effective and to make the most efficient use of scarce resources. When a death is anticipated, not only the patient, but also his/her family can be prepared appropriately well before the event. This is shown to reduce anxiety, depression and post-traumatic stress disorder among the bereaved family.

Appendix

Sequential Organ Failure Assessment score (SOFA score), is used to track a person's status during the stay in an intensive care unit (ICU) to determine the extent of a person's organ function or rate of failure. The score is based on six different scores, one each for the respiratory, cardiovascular, hepatic, coagulation, renal and neurological systems.

PaO_2/FiO_2 (mm Hg)	*SOFA score*	
<400	1	
<300	2	
<200 and mechanically ventilated	3	
<100 and mechanically ventilated	4	
Glasgow Coma Scale	*SOFA score*	
13–14	1	
10–12	2	
6–9	3	
<6	4	
Mean arterial pressure or administration of vasopressors required		*SOFA score*
MAP <70 mm Hg		1
Dop ≤5 or dob (any dose)		2
Dop >5 or epi ≤0.1 or nor ≤0.1		3
Dop >15 or epi >0.1 or nor >0.1		4

(vasopressor drug doses are in µg/kg/min)

Abbreviations: Dop, dopamine; Dob, dobutamine; Epi, epinephrine; Nor, norepinephrine.

Bilirubin (mg/dL) (µmol/L)	*SOFA score*
1.2–1.9 (> 20–32)	1
2.0–5.9 (33–101)	2
6.0–11.9 (102–204)	3
>12.0 (>204)	4

If bilirubin is less than 1.2, the score is 0

Platelets × 10^3/µL	*SOFA score*
<150	1
<100	2
<50	3
<20	4

If platelet is more than 150 then score is 0

Creatinine (mg/dL) (µmol/L) (or urine output)	*SOFA score*
1.2–1.9 (110–170)	1
2.0–3.4 (171–299)	2
3.5–4.9 (300–440) (or <500 mL/d)	3
>5.0 (>440) (or <200 mL/d)	4

The APACHE II Severity of Disease Classification System

Physiologic variable	+4		+3	+2	+1	0	+1	+2	+3	+4
Temperature-rectal (°C)	≥41		32–40.9		38.5–38.9	36–38.4	34–35.9	32–33.9	30–31.9	≤29.9
Mean arterial pressure (mm Hg)	≥160		130–159	110–129		70–109		50–59		≤49
Heart rate	≥180		140–179	110–139		70–109		55–69	40–54	≤39
Respiratory rate (nonventilated or ventilated)	≥50		35–49		25–34	12–24	10–11	6–9		≤5
Oxygenation (mm Hg) a. FiO_2 >0, 5 use $A\text{-}aDO_2$ b. FiO_2 <0, 5 use PaO_2	a	≥500	350–499	200–349		<200				
	b					>70	61–70		55–60	<55
Arterial pH	≥7.7		7.6–7.69		7.5–7.59	7.33–7.49		7.25–7.32	7.15–7.24	<7.15
Serum sodium (mmol/L)	≥180		160–179	155–159	150–154	130–149		120–129	111–119	≤110
Serum potassium (mmol/L)	≥7		6–6.9		5.5–5.9	3.5–5.4	3–3.4	2.5–2.9		<2.5
Serum creatinine (mg/dL, double point score for acute renal failure)	≥3.5		2–3.4	1.5–1.9		0.6–1.4		<0.6		
Hematocrit (%)	≥60			50–59.9	46–49.9	30–45.9		20–29.9		<20

Contd...

Contd...

White blood count (in 1000/mm²)	≥40		20–39.9	15–19.9	3–14.9		1–2.9		<1
Glasgow Coma Scale (GCS)	Score = 15 minus actual GCS								
Serum HCO_3 (venous, mmol/L, use if no ABGs)	≥52	41–51.9		32–40.9	22–31.9		18–21.9	15–17.9	<15
A = Total acute physiology score APS	Sum of the 12 individual variable points								
B = Age points ≤44 years 0 points 45–54 years 2 points 55–64 years 3 points 65–74 years 5 points ≥75 years 6 points	*C = Chronic health points* If the patient has a history of severe organ system insufficiency or is immunocompromised assign points as follows: a. For nonoperative or emergency postoperative patients—5 points b. For elective postoperative patients—2 points								
APACHE II Score = Sum of A (APS points) + B (Age points) + C (Chronic health points)									

Source: Knaus WA, Draper EA, Wagner DP, Zimmerman JE. APACHE II: a severity of disease classification system. Crit Care Med. 1985;13(10):818-29.

Normal Arterial Blood Gas Values

Normal ABG Values

- pH: 7.35–7.45
- PCO_2: 35–45 mm Hg
- PO_2: >80 mm Hg
- HCO_3: 22–28 mEq/L

Arterial Blood Gasses and Compensatory Mechanisms

Normal Value	*pH: 7.35–7.45*	*PCO2: 35–45 mm Hg*	*$NaHCO_3$: 22–28 mm Hg/L*	*Compensation*
Respiratory Alkalosis	Up	Down	Normal until compensation	Kidneys will decrease $NaHCO_3$. (slow)
Respiratory Acidosis	Down	Up	Normal until compensation	Kidneys will retain $NaHCO_3$. (slow)
Metabolic Alkalosis	Up	Normal until compensation	Up	Lungs will try to increase pCO_2 by hypoventilation
Metabolic Acidosis	Down	Normal until compensation	Down	Lungs will try to decrease pCO_2 by hyperventilation

Index

Page numbers followed by *f* refer to figure and *t* refer to table.

A

Acetylcholine 44
Acid/base disturbance 90
Acquired immune deficiency syndrome 174
Acquired thrombophilias 34
Adenovirus 111
Agitation 30
Agranular leukocytes 94
Airborne precautions 112
Airway
- assessment 9
- electively, steps in securing 11
- interventions 9, 10
- lower 9
- maintain 142
- management 9, 13
  - elective 11
- obstruction, causes of 10*t*
- patency 9
- positive pressure, continuous 82
- pressure 30
- protection 149

Albumin 96
Allen's test, modified 62
Allergic reactions 90
Ambient air 9, 10
American College of Cardiology 223
American College of Critical Care Medicine 189
American Heart Association 222, 223
American Nurses Association 214
Amikacin 172
Analgesia 31, 33, 50
- therapy 50

Analgesics 13, 28
Anaphylactoid reaction 126
Aneurysm 130
- false 132

Angiotensinogen converting enzyme 126
Antacids 37
Antiarrhythmics 126
Antibiotic
- assays 172
- levels of 172*t*

Anticipated difficult airway, assessment for 12*t*
Anticoagulation protocols 139
Aortic dissection 129
Aortic end diastolic pressure 133
Aortic regurgitation, severe 129
Aortoiliac disease, severe 130
Aplastic anemia 95
Arrhythmias 29
Arterial blood gas 74, 78, 230
- values, normal 230

Arterial cannulation 62
Arterial catheter 61
Arterial partial pressure of oxygen 76
Arterial pressure
- mean 146, 158
- waveforms, abnormal 62

Arterial pulse contour analysis 59
Arterial waveforms 63*f*
- components of 62

Arteriovenous fistula 132
Artifacts 68*f*
Asthma 29
Atrial arrhythmias 139
Atrial fibrillation 221
Atrial flutter 221
Atropine 126

B

Bacterial culture 169
Balanced liquid nutrition, complete 101
- isotonic 101

Balloon aortic end diastolic pressure 132
Balloon pump timing 131
Barotrauma 30
Basophils 94
Bedside cardiovascular ultrasound 118
Benzodiazepines 52
Biomedical waste management 180

Bitemporal syndrome 46
Bleeding 95
Blood 93
  culture 166, 170
    bottle, aerobic 167
    bottle, anaerobic 167
    collection 167
    number of 166
    timing of 166
    volume of 166
  for virology 1786
  functions of 93
  glucose, normal 38
  pressure 58, 78, 126
    mean 133
  products 93, 96*t*
    administration of 96
Bloodstream infections bundle, catheter-related 31
Body tissue cells 73
Bordetella pertussis 111
Bowel care 31, 39
Braden scale 25*t*
Braden scoring form 209*f*
Bradycardia 34, 126
Brain injury
  compressive 146
  primary 145
  secondary 146
Breath cycle, levels in 70*f*
Breathing 74, 137
  coordination 47
  exercises, deep 29
  trial 39
Bronchial hygiene 29
Bronchiectasis 28
Bronchitis, chronic 28
Bronchospasm 29
Brucella 165
Burns 37

C

Calcium hypochlorite 185
Calories 32
Canadian Standards Association 187
Capnogram 70*f*
Carbon dioxide 73
  end tidal 69
  monitoring, end tidal 67, 69
Cardiac arrest 221
Cardiac output 58
  monitoring 59
Cardiac structures 66
Cardiac surgery, complications after 139
Cardiac tamponade 140
Cardiopulmonary
  bypass 136
  resuscitation 70
    documentation 209
Cardiovascular
  life support, advanced 222
  status 149
Catheter
  specimens 168
  types of 103
Central alpha-agonists 53
Central nervous system 145
Central venous
  access, complications of 66
  catheter 64
  oxygen saturation 118
  pressure 57, 64, 118, 136
    components of 65*f*
    waves 64
Cerebral edema 152
Cerebrospinal fluid 166, 171
Cerebrovascular accidents 147
Charting, types of 201
Chemical disinfectants 187
Chemical prophylaxis 35
Chemical waste 180
Chest physiotherapy 28
  techniques for 29
Chickenpox 112
Chloramine 185
Chlorhexidine skin antisepsis 115
Clostridium difficile 39, 40
  enterocolitis 37
Clotting factor deficiency 96
Clotting problems 90
Coagulation disorders 95
Coagulopathy 99
Colloid osmotic pressure 94
Communication barriers 18
Communication, barriers in 192*t*
Complete balanced liquid nutrition, high-calorie 101
Congestive cardiac failure 29
Congestive heart failure 82
Conjunctiva 19
Consciousness, level of 142
Copious secretions 28
Coronary angiography 126
Coronary artery
  bypass graft 136
  disease 125
Coronary syndrome, acute 125
Cortisol excess 44

Cough reflex 15
Cranial nerve examination 142
Critical care medicine 190*f*
Critical result intimation 194
Cryoprecipitate 96
Cystic fibrosis 28
Cytomegalovirus 146

D

Daily oral care with chlorhexidine 114
Daily sedation interruption 39
Damping, effect of 63*f*
Defibrillation 221
Delirium 42
- diagnosis of 45*f*
- in intensive care unit 42
- management of 46*f*
- monitoring, management 47
- outcomes 43*f*
- pathogenesis of 44*f*
- prevention of 47
- types of 43*t*

Dementia 46
Dexmedetomidine 34, 48
Diabetes mellitus 127
Diarrhea 39
- antibiotic-associated 39
- reasons for 102

Diastolic blood pressure 59
- higher 62

Dilutional coagulopathy 96
Disinfectants, dilutions of 185*t*
Disseminated intravascular coagulopathy 95
Dopamine 44
Drug 3, 138
- allergy 38
- doses 127
- for intubation 14*t*
- selection of 33

Dyshemoglobinemia 69

E

Echocardiography 59, 126, 136
Ejection fraction 58
Electrocardiography, continuous 78
Electroencephalogram 48
Electrolyte disturbance 90
Elemental diets 101
Elevated intracranial pressure 52, 141
Emergency unresponsive patients 11
End-diastolic volume 58
Endotracheal aspirations 170
Endotracheal tubes 108
End-systolic volume 58
Enteral feeds 38
Environment, maintain safe 148
Environmental cleaning 112
Environmental control 110
Eosinophils 94
Erythrocytes 93
Esomeprazole 37
Esophageal varices 99
European Pressure Advisory Panel 23
Expiration ratio 74, 75
Extubation 9, 12
Eye
- care 19, 21
  - practices, existing 21
- physiology, altered 20
- problems, common 21
- protection 110

Eyelid closure 19, 22

F

Face shield 110
Fast flush test 63, 64*f*
Feeding 31
- complications of enteral 102
- contraindication of enteral 99
- duration of enteral 99
- tube with tape 100*f*

Fentanyl 14
First aid 176
First morning sputum 170
Fluid 138
- administration, route of 90
- in body, distribution of 87
- management in burns 91
- overload 140
- replacement therapy 87
- therapy, complications of 90

Flush solution 60
Fondaparinux 36
Forced expiratory techniques 29
Fractures 37
Fresh frozen plasma 93, 95, 95*t*, 155
Fungal culture 169, 170
Fungal examinations 170

G

Gamma-aminobutyric acid 44
Gases into circulation, transport of 73
Gastric 99
- lavage 172

residual volume 32
tolerance 32
Gastrointestinal bleed 99
Gastrointestinal infections 171
Gastrointestinal prophylaxis 114
Gastrointestinal samples 171
Gastrointestinal tract, functioning 98
Genotoxic waste 180
Gentamicin 172
Glasgow coma scale 141, 142*t*
Glomerular filtration rate 155
Gloves 110
Glycemic control 31, 38
Gown 110
Granular leukocytes 94
Gut functions 99

H

Haemophilus influenzae 111, 169
Hemorrhage, intracranial 147
Haloperidol 48
Hand hygiene 109, 114
five moments for 116*f*
Hand wash, procedure for 116*f*
Hazardous waste, classification of 179
Head injury 37
Head of bed elevation 113
Heart failure 127
management of 126
Hematoma 132
Hemodynamic 57
disturbance 30
monitoring, steps of 59
Hemoglobin 93
Hemoptysis, severe 29
Hepatic encephalopathy 153, 153*t*
Hepatic failure 37
fulminant 151
Hepatitis
B 176
exposure to 176
C 176
exposure to 177
virus infection 174
Hepatopulmonary syndrome 154
Hepatorenal syndrome 155
Herpes simplex virus 145
Herpes zoster 112
Hormone replacement therapy 34
Hospital waste
categories 182
management of 179
Hospital-acquired pressure ulcer 24
Human immunodeficiency virus 176, 177
post-exposure prophylaxis 177
test 174
Hygiene, maintain personal 142
Hypercoagulability 34
Hypercoagulation 34
Hyperglycemia 38
Hyperinflation 29
Hyperkalemia 90
Hypocalcemia 37, 90
Hypomagnesemia 37
Hyponatremia 90
Hypotension 76, 80, 154
Hypothermia 90
Hypotonic solutions 92
Hypoxemia 30, 76
Hypoxia 80

I

Ill-patients, acutely 89
Incentive spirometry 29
Indwelling catheter removal 31, 40
Infection 105, 107, 156
control 3
Control Program 109
Infectious diseases, serologic diagnosis of 172
Infectious waste 179
Inflammatory mediators 44
Influenza virus 111
Inspiration 74, 75
Inspiratory flow rate 74, 75
Inspired oxygen concentration 74
Intensive care unit 15, 20, 23, 28, 31, 42, 50, 98, 100, 107, 157, 197, 204*f*, 206*f*
bundles 113
physiotherapy in 28
team 137
Intercostals drains 40
Interfaces 83
Intermittent mandatory ventilation 75
Intra-aortic balloon pump 128, 129*f*, 136
Intracranial pressure 28
concept of rising 143
monitoring 154
Invasive arterial pressure monitoring 62

Invasive hemodynamic monitoring system 60
Invasive strategy 128
Isbar tool 193
Isocal 101
Isolation precautions 111

J

Joint Commission for Accreditation for Healthcare Organization 214, 219

K

Kidney
- function tests 48
- injury, acute 92, 154

L

Laxatives 39
Leukemia 95
Leukocytes 94
Linen 110
Liver 151
- dysfunction 151
- failure 151
  - acute 151, 152, 156*t*
- transplantation 156, 156*t*

Lobar atelectasis, acute 28
Lumbar puncture 48
Lung injury, acute 76
Lymphocytes 94

M

Magnacal 101
Mask 110
Measles 112
Mechanical devices 35
Mechanical tricuspid 66
Mechanical ventilation 28, 71, 73, 74, 76
Mental status 142
Metabolic acidosis 230
Metabolic alkalosis 230
Midazolam 14
Minimally invasive cardiac surgery 136
Molecular weight heparin, low 35
Monitoring during mechanical ventilation 78
Monocytes 94
Motor system 142
Multiple organ dysfunction syndrome 57
Muscle disease 127
Mycobacterial culture 169, 170
Mycobacterium tuberculosis 112, 165
Mycoplasma pneumonia 111
Myocardial infarction, management of uncomplicated acute 125
Myocarditis 127

N

Na hypochlorite powder 185
N-acetylcysteine 159
Nail polish 69
Nasal swabs 169
Nasopharyngeal suction 169
Nasopharyngeal swabs 169
National Institute for Health and Care Excellence 30
National pressure ulcer advisory panel 23
Needlestick injury 174
Neisseria meningitides 111, 169
Nephrotic syndrome 34
Nephrotoxins 158
Neurocritical care 141
Neurological diseases 76
Neurological emergencies 141
Neurological examination 142
Neurological injury 28
Neuromuscular blocking agents 13
Neurotransmitter mechanism 44
Neutral amino acid 44
Neutrophils 94
Newer agents 36
Nonconvulsive status epilepticus 46
Noninvasive positive-pressure ventilation 82
Noninvasive ventilation 82, 83
Non-opioids 34
Nonpharmacological management 48
Non-ST elevated myocardial infarction 125
Nonsteroid anti-inflammatory drugs 34, 50, 126, 158
Normothermia, maintaining 138
Nucleic acid amplification 172
Nurses, role of 3, 66, 69
Nursing
- care plans 206*f*
- communication in intensive care units 189
- documentation, computerized 217

initial assessment form 202f
management 147
progress notes 205f
Nutrition 26
enteral 98
high-nitrogen liquid 101
therapy 37
Nutritional assessment 98
Nutritional delivery, assessing 104
Nutritional support
enteral 98
in critical care 98
route of 98

O

Observe vital signs 142
Obstacles, mechanical 17
Obstructive pulmonary disease, chronic 75, 76, 78, 82, 224
Occipital syndrome 46
Ocular surgery 29
Opioid 33, 50
administration techniques 50
Optimal catheter site selection 115
Optimal hemodynamics 37
Oral
assessment 16
care
in intensive care unit 15
practices 16
colonization 15
cultures 169
feeding 32
phosphorous supplements 39
care 15, 17
Organ
donation 212
transplantation 37
Osmolite 101
Osteoporosis 29
Oxidative metabolism 44
Oxygen
concentration 74
saturation 67

P

Packed cells 93
Packed red cell transfusion 95t
Paddle placement 222
Pain scales 33
Pantoprazole 37
Parenteral nutrition 32, 98
support 103
Parkland formula, modified 92
Partial thromboplastin time, activated 96
Patency 9
Pathological waste 179
Perfusion state, low 69
Peripheral vascular disease 130
Permit lung healing 74
Personal protective equipment 109
Pharmaceutical
containing 180
waste 180
Pharmacological management 48
Phlebostatic axis 61f
Plasma 94
proteins 94
Platelet 94, 95
apheresis 95
from apheresis donation 95t
loss, increased 95
rich plasma 95
Pleural effusions 140
Pneumonia 28, 37, 38
Pneumothorax 29, 30, 140
Polyethylene covers 22
Positive end expiratory pressure 70, 74, 75, 78
Posttraumatic stress disorder 33
Potassium chloride syrup 39
Potential eye problems 20
Pregnancy 34
Prepyloric feeding 99
Pressure 65
bag 60
control 77
sore 23, 149
transducer 60
tubing 60
ulcer 23
Pressure-regulated volume control 77
Prophylactic therapies 159
Prophylaxis
post-exposure 176
primary 35
secondary 35
Propofol 14, 52
Prothrombin time 96
Proton pump inhibitors 37
Pseudomonas aeruginosa 16
Pulmonary artery 57
catheter 59, 65

Pulmonary capillary wedge pressure 138
Pulmonary disease
  chronic 28
  restrictive 28
Pulmonary edema 29, 90
Pulmonary embolism 34
Pulmonary embolus 29
Pulmonary gas exchange 74
Pulmonary system, physiology of 73
Pulmonary thromboembolism 127
Pulmonary valves 66
Pulmonary vascular resistance 58
Pulse 221
  oximetry 67, 68, 78
Pulseless ventricular tachycardia 221
Pupil
  reaction 142
  size 142

R

Rabeprazole 37
Ramsay sedation scale 51*t*
Ranitidine 37
Rectal swabs 172
Recumbancy 28
Red blood cells 93
Rehabilitation 148
Relieve respiratory distress 74
Renal disease, end stage 127
Renal failure 37
  acute 157
Renal replacement therapy 154, 157, 159
Respiratory
  acidosis 230
  alkalosis 230
  arrest 76
  compromise 154
  distress syndrome, acute 78, 102
  drive 9, 10
  failure 140
    acute 28
  muscle fatigue, reverse 74
  samples 169
  syndrome, severe acute 111
  tract samples, lower 170
Resuscitation 87
Rhinovirus 111
Rib fracture 29
Richmond agitation-sedation scale 45
Right ventricle 57
Riker sedation-agitation scale 51
Rocuronium 14
Rubella virus 112

S

Salvage 88
Securing tube 99
Sedation 31
  assessment 51
  in critically ill 50
  therapy 52
Sedative 28
  agents 47
Sensory system 142
Sepsis 34, 37
  bundle 116
Shock 37
Skin, disinfection of 167
Skull fracture, base of 99
Sodium hypochlorite 185
Spinal cord injury 37
Spinal injury 149
Spontaneous awakening 39
Spontaneous breathing trial 31, 39
Staphylococcus aureus 16, 107, 169
Stasis 34
Status epilepticus 150
St-elevated myocardial infarction 125
Sterile body fluids 171
Sterilization 113, 179
Sternal wound infection 140
Streptococcus pneumoniae 169
Streptococcus pyogenes 172
Stress-related mucosal injury 81
Stroke 147
  volume 57
    index 58
Sucralfate-mucosal protective agent 37
Sun downing 46
Swan gang pulmonary artery 126
Synchronized cardioversion 126
Synchronized intermittent mandatory ventilation 77
Systemic capillary bed 73
Systemic inflammatory response syndrome 34
Systemic vascular resistance 58
Systolic blood pressure 59, 62, 133
Systolic pressure, assisted peak 132

T

Tachycardia, supraventricular 221
Tear formation 19
Temporoparietal syndrome 46
Throat swabs 169
Thrombocytes 94
Thrombocytopenia 95
Thrombolysis, early 126
Thrombolytic therapy
  arrhythmias, complication of 126
Thromboprophylaxis 31, 34, 35
Tidal volume 74
Tissue
  donation 212
  injury, deep 24
  plasminogen activator 145
  samples 170, 171
Tobramycin 172
Total body water, distribution of 88*f*
Total parenteral nutrition solution 103
Toxin 172
Tracheal stimulation 29, 30
Tracheostomy 170
Transpulmonary thermodilution 59
Trauma 34, 127
Traumatic brain injury 32, 144
Tube care 100
Tube management 99
Tube placement 99
Tube position inside abdomen 100*f*
Tubular necrosis, acute 154, 157

U

Ulcer prophylaxis 31, 37
Undrained pneumothorax 28
Unfractionated heparin 35
Unique hospital identification 193
Upper airway 9
Upper gastrointestinal surgery 99
Upper respiratory tract samples 169
Urinary tract infection, catheter-associated 115
Urine 167

V

Valve
  dysfunction 126
  surgery 139
Vancomycin 172
Vancomycin-resistant enterococci 172
Varicella zoster virus 112
Vascular access device 194
Vascular endothelial injury 34
Vein thrombosis, deep 34, 113, 208*f*
Venous foot pumps 35
Venous oxygen saturation 66
Venous thromboembolism 34, 81
Venovenous hemodialysis, continuous 154
Ventilation 73
  artificial 15
  dual-modes of 78
  modes of 77
Ventilator
  mode 74
  rate 75
  settings 74
  troubleshooting 79
Ventilator-associated pneumonia 15, 31, 81
  bundle 31, 113
Ventricular fibrillation 126, 221
Ventricular septal defect 126
Ventricular tachycardia 126, 221
Viral culture 169

W

Ward function 4
Washing hands with soap and water, procedure for 117*f*
Waste
  management 179
  type of 182, 183
  with heavy metals 180
White blood cells 94
World Heath Organization 116*f*
Wound swabs 170